GROWING HAPPY, HEALTHY YOUNG MINDS

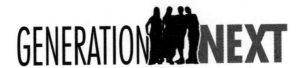

GENERATION NEXT

GROWING HAPPY, HEALTHY YOUNG MINDS

Ed. DR RAMESH MANOCHA
WITH GYONGYI HORVATH

ROBINSON

ROBINSON

First published in Australia and New Zealand in 2017 by Hachette Australia

First published in Great Britain in 2018 by Robinson

A CIP catalogue record for this book
is available from the British Library.

ISBN: 978-1-47214-194-1

Printed and bound in Great Britain by CPI Group (UK) Ltd, Croydon CR0 4YY

Papers used by Robinson are from well-managed forests
and other responsible sources

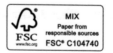

Robinson
An imprint of
Little, Brown Book Group
Carmelite House
50 Victoria Embankment
London EC4Y 0DZ

An Hachette UK Company
www.hachette.co.uk

www.improvementzone.co.uk.

Foreword   ix
    Andrew Fuller

How to Use this Book   xii
    Dr Ramesh Manocha & Gyongyi Horvath

Where to Get Help   xvi

HOW TO HELP   1

1. Helping Young People Get Help for Mental Health Problems   3
   Debra Rickwood

2. What to do in a Mental Health Crisis   17
   Dr Claire Kelly

COMMON MENTAL HEALTH CONCERNS   33

3. Bullying Basics   35
   Sandra Craig

4. Anxiety in Young People   53
   Professor Jennie Hudson & Dr Anna McKinnon

5. Depression in Young People   64
   Dr Bridianne O'Dea & Dr Aliza Werner-Seidler

6. Understanding Self-harm   80
   Dr Claire Kelly

7. Suicide and Attempted Suicide   96
   Dr Claire Kelly

8. Towards Prevention: Understanding Child Sexual Assault   114
   Carol Ronken

ALCOHOL AND DRUGS 131

9. Talking About Alcohol and Drugs 133
Siobhan Lawler, Nicola Newton, Katrina Champion & Lexine Stapinski

10. Supporting a Young Person in their Decision
Not to Use Alcohol or Other Drugs 150
Paul Dillon

11. Teens, Parties and Alcohol: A Practical Guide
to Keeping Them Safe 166
Paul Dillon

BODY IMAGE AND EATING DISORDERS 179

12. Understanding Eating Disorders in Young People 181
Dr Tina Peckmezian, Dr Michelle Blanchard & Danielle Cuthbert

13. Excessive Dieting and Exercise 202
Amy Burton, Andreea Heriseanu, Brooke Donnelly & Phillip Aouad

14. Anorexia Nervosa 217
Brooke Donnelly, Phillip Aouad, Amy Burton & Andreea Heriseanu

15. Bulimia and Binge Eating 233
Andreea Heriseanu, Brooke Donnelly, Amy Burton & Phillip Aouad

16. Bigorexia: Muscle Dysmorphia in Young People 250
Dr Scott Griffiths

17. Fostering a Positive Body Image 265
Professor Susan Paxton & Dr Siân McLean

RESILIENCE, POSITIVE PSYCHOLOGY AND A HEALTHY LIFESTYLE 279

18. What is Resilience and How to Do It 281
Andrew Fuller

19. Harnessing the Minecraft Mindset for Success 292
Dan Haesler

20. Using Positive Psychology 306
Dr Justin Coulson

21. Food, Mood and Mental Health 323
Felice Jacka

22. Understanding the Teenage Brain   335
    Dr Michael Nagel

23. Online Time Management   349
    Tena Davies

Endnotes   359

The Mental Stillness App   364
    Kabir Sattarshetty

FOREWORD

A friend once told me that the introduction is always the least-read part of any book. 'It's always skipped over as people rush to get to what you have to say,' she said. 'Never,' she advised, 'never waste your time writing an introduction!'

So here I am, living proof that advice may be listened to but is rarely followed.

The experience of many young people is that growing up is a bit like going on a wild roller-coaster ride. The aim of this book is to inform you so that you can help as many young people as possible to stay in the trolley car and not fall on the tracks.

From my days working in mental health crisis teams, I recall a wild-eyed young man I visited at home. I started to talk to him in the back of his garden while he swung a machete back and forth. The machete looked sharp. As he looked at me with fear and desperation in his eyes, my overriding thought was, *What the hell do I do now?* In my career, this question has returned to me many times.

While many of the mental health challenges that we and the young people we care for will not be as extreme as this, the situation illustrates how out of our depth we can feel when trying to help a young person in their moment of need. Although no single book can tell you exactly what to do now, or next, *Growing Happy, Healthy Young Minds* goes a long way towards helping. It contains sweat, fear, hope, dreams and the methods and experiences of many skilled experts to help you.

As I stood in that garden, the trickle of fear on the back of my neck told me I had only one chance to get it right. With every young person we work with, we also often get only one chance to change things to a positive direction. That single opportunity, if taken, can have powerful effects. Effects that can last a lifetime.

This book will be important to anyone who is the parent of a young person or has an interest in working with people aged under twenty-five, such as youth workers, school support workers, social workers, child protection workers, psychologists, community workers, therapists, teachers and year-level coordinators. The type of work they do is variously described as counselling, assisting, mentoring, therapy and even 'hanging around with'.

This book is a bit like a single ride on a roller-coaster. We know we have only one chance to help parents and care givers and we want to get it right. I suspect you will delve into this book as you need, picking up topics as they relate to young people in your family or who you are working with.

Every chapter of this book deals with an issue that, if tackled properly, can change a young person's life for the better. In some cases those chapters will not only be life-changing but quite possibly lifesaving.

We are proud of the accumulated wisdom collected in *Growing Happy, Healthy Young Minds* and even more excited about how you might be able to use it to open possibilities in the lives of the young people you work with.

On behalf of all of the clinicians, I would like to thank our teachers, especially those of you who thought you were our clients.

I would also like to thank the team at Generation Next: Dr Ramesh and Mrs Gita Manocha, Gyongyi Horvath, Ning Pruttivarasin, Bronte Baskin, Lisa Evans, Nick Chuah, Natalie Vo, Blake Galera-Holliss, Neil Harris, John Towner, Christie Ho, Shari Borodkin, Kimberley Thomas and many others who have worked to support the development of this book.

Most importantly we need to acknowledge the team at Hachette Australia: Fiona Hazard, Publishing Director, and Sophie Hamley, publisher, for their wisdom in recognising the need for a book like this; Sophie Hamley and Sophie Mayfield for going above and beyond the call of duty to get this information out for the benefit of young people.

Each year Generation Next, as a not-for-profit charitable organisation, works to increase the skills and knowledge of many thousands of professionals and young people through its face-to-face events, live webcasts and free online resources. In doing so, it helps us all to create a better world for our next-generation leaders to inherit.

Andrew Fuller
Melbourne, 2017

HOW TO USE THIS BOOK

Growing Happy, Healthy Young Minds is designed to be read in separate bites. When you are concerned about a certain issue, look up the relevant chapter and read it. Each chapter is self-contained and does not assume that you have read any other section of the book. At the end of each chapter useful resources are included for you to access if you want more in-depth information, including resources, websites, articles and books, along with listing other chapters within this book that cover related issues to your main concern.

Growing Happy, Healthy Young Minds also has an excellent supporting website which you can access via www.generationnext.com.au – click on the book icon. Click on a chapter title and you will be taken to a page that will contain:

- Author photos, bios and books and articles written by them.
- Where available the author's own website, in case you want to get in touch directly with them.
- Further reading, websites and resources with hyperlinks wherever possible.
- Where provided, the references used by the authors to write their chapters.
- Links to relevant lectures, interviews and short educational clips from the Generation Next YouTube channel.
- Updates to chapters as new developments and advances occur.

To continue to stay up to date on information and developments in this important field, you can also:

- Subscribe to the free weekly Generation Next newsletter, which provides a range of interesting news and information curated from around the world concerning the mental health and wellbeing of young people.
- Read the Generation Next blog, join our Facebook community and follow us on Twitter.
- Subscribe to our YouTube Channel to receive a new video in your inbox each week.
- Attend one of our one-day seminars that are listed on our website.

USE THIS BOOK TO HELP OTHERS!

Are you a parent?

- Give a copy of this book to your child's grandparents, aunties and uncles.
- Buy a copy for your child's school or teacher.
- Encourage your school's PTA to host an event for fellow parents, focusing on youth mental health using resources and content from the book.
- Provide relevant sections of the book to your teen (recommended fourteen years +) to increase mental health literacy.
- Use strategies and tips from the book to start conversations about tricky topics with your child/teen about issues affecting them.
- Use the resources directly to create a support services index to raise awareness of help-seeking avenues that you can post on your fridge – this can help your child/teen and can be used by them to help their friends.
- Recommend the book to others in your parent or community groups.
- Share the book with other parents or anyone who is concerned about a young person.

Are you a teacher or teacher-in-training?

- Recommend this book to parents in your school community.
- Read chapters as part of your ongoing professional development and learning.
- Host professional development sessions for colleagues at school using content from the book to improve individual and organisational professional practice.
- Use some of the content for a mental-health-themed parent–teacher event, e.g. recognising common mental health concerns.
- Use relevant chapters in your lesson plans to meet relevant curriculum requirements (e.g. in PSHE).
- Pick an issue covered in the book and encourage your students to do a project or a peer-education initiative around it.
- Get the Student Representative Council or school to pick an issue(s) from the book and run a peer-education programme or an awareness day around it.
- Use the resources directly to create a support services index for your class or school to raise awareness of help-seeking avenues and so that students and staff know where they can go for help.
- Share warning signs and red flags about particular issues with parents of students you are concerned about.
- Use content to shape school wellbeing programmes, including induction programmes for new students and year levels.
- Use content from the book's supporting website (like videos and podcasts) for further professional development and learning.
- Order copies for your school library.

Are you a professional working with young people?

- Read chapters as part of your ongoing professional development and learning.
- Use some of the content for in-house professional development sessions for colleagues to improve individual and organisational professional practice.

- Share relevant content when working with young people or their parents, in particular relating to warning signs and red flags.
- Use the resources directly to create a support services index to raise awareness of help-seeking avenues that can be shared at work and put up in common areas.
- Use content from the supporting website (videos and podcasts) for further professional development and learning.
- Pick an issue and use the book's recommended resources to undertake further professional learning.
- Pick an issue and use the book's content as a springboard for undertaking research to improve the impact of your work with young people.
- Use content of the book to help inform your organisation's mental health policy/plan.
- Order copies for your organisation's library.

Advocate for a greater focus on mental health and help create environments that are supportive of young people's wellbeing.

Dr Ramesh Manocha & Gyongyi Horvath

WHERE TO GET HELP

If you or a young person you know needs to talk to someone anonymously, or needs help, the following services are available.

Samaritans

Samaritans operates a twenty-four-hour confidential telephone counselling line and information service, and can provide contact details for other help services.

Helpline: 116 123 (free)
Email: jo@samaritans.org
Hours: Helpline is available 24/7, 365 days a year

Childline

Childline operates a twenty-four-hour confidential telephone and online counselling service for anyone under the age of nineteen in the UK.

Helpline: 0800 1111 (free)
Online counselling and email: www.childline.org.uk
Hours: Helpline is available 24/7, 365 days a year

Emergencies

999 or 112

HOW TO HELP

Helping Young People Get Help for Mental Health Problems   3

What to do in a Mental Health Crisis   17

1. HELPING YOUNG PEOPLE GET HELP FOR MENTAL HEALTH PROBLEMS

Debra Rickwood

Young people are at the highest risk of mental health problems, yet are the least likely to reach out for help. This means that the adults in their lives need to be ready, willing and able to support them to get the help they need when they need it. Enabling young people to get appropriate support as early as possible will help reduce the impact of mental ill health on their lives.

INTRODUCTION

Mental health problems are common during the teenage years, as this is the time when many such issues first become evident. While behavioural and some anxiety disorders generally start during childhood, it is in the teenage years that depression, self-harm, suicidal thoughts, substance use, disordered eating and eating disorders, and mood disorders emerge. In late adolescence and early adulthood, psychosis begins to occur. In any given year, it is estimated that about one-quarter of young people in Australia aged sixteen to twenty-four years will have a diagnosable mental health problem. By age twenty-one, just over half of all young people will have experienced a clinically significant mental health disorder.

Because mental health issues are so common, there is a tendency to consider them an inevitable part of the transition from childhood to adulthood. The period of adolescence has long been viewed as a time of 'storm and stress', which needs to be endured and survived by all involved – the adolescents themselves as well as those around them. But this view condemns many young people and their families to, at best, painful psychological distress and, at worst, a downward trajectory into long-term mental ill health and associated poor social and vocational outcomes. Appropriate recognition of and effective responses to adolescent mental health problems are critical – and comprise an essential responsibility for caring adults in young people's lives.

WHY DON'T WE INTERVENE?

Adults can be reluctant to intervene even when they are concerned about a young person's mental wellbeing, and there are many good reasons for this. The first is that we tend to attribute concerning changes in behaviour to the nature of adolescence itself. We see many potential symptoms of mental health problems – moodiness, withdrawal, irritability, lack of organisation – as just part and parcel of puberty, raging hormones, adolescent angst … and we hope that the phase will soon pass. It is hard to know when something is really wrong, and when it's a temporary concern that will sort itself out. It is certainly difficult to judge which issues will resolve without intervention and which ones are indications of something more serious that warrants attention.

Another reason we don't intervene is fear of making things worse and creating a problem when there needn't be one. In particular, we don't want to 'medicalise' or 'pathologise' components of the human condition. Given mental health issues are so common during the teen years, it is easy to take the view that we should accept many symptoms as inevitable for this life stage and expect young people to be sufficiently resilient to survive.

Further, in Britain, as elsewhere, many of us have a strongly held value to mind our own business and not interfere in other people's lives. As a result, we turn a blind eye to issues that might concern us, avoid speaking up and intervening, and hope that people can sort out their own problems.

From a more constructive viewpoint, many adults are reluctant to intervene in order to support and respect young people's growing autonomy. We understand that they want and need to learn to sort things out for themselves and stand on their own. It is hard to know when and how to intervene in a way that respects and facilitates young people's independence, resilience and own problem-solving capabilities.

There is growing concern about the predominance of 'helicopter' and 'lawnmower' parenting, where all problems are anticipated and removed. This approach is certainly not advocated; it is essential for the development of a strong personal identity and resilient emerging adulthood that teenagers are progressively enabled to manage their own lives, including resolving their own problems and making their own decisions (including making mistakes), when appropriate and as safety and maturity allows.

WHY WE SHOULD INTERVENE

Despite these understandable barriers to getting involved, there are stronger arguments for doing so, when warranted. Fundamentally, mental health problems are far from benign and can cause serious damage at this critical formative stage of life. While they are prevalent and some will resolve without intervention, most mental health problems are associated with considerable distress and can seriously harm social relationships and emotional and cognitive development, as well as educational, personal and vocational achievements. Minor problems may progress to more serious mental disorders, can often accumulate additional issues (such as substance use), and are likely to recur if not effectively treated. A growing body of evidence shows that not intervening, or delaying effective intervention, exacerbates issues and leads to poorer outcomes. Although psychology and psychiatry are fields where there is much yet to discover, there is a great deal that is currently understood about how to alleviate distress and treat the symptoms of mental ill health, and effective interventions are available.

Regardless of their growing maturity, young people are not well equipped to help themselves, so they need the concerned adults in their lives to step up to this responsibility. To start with, young people tend not to recognise mental health issues; they ignore and minimise symptoms, hope they will go away, or think they are just part of growing up. If they do recognise that things aren't quite right, they often don't have a language or way to convey this to other people. They are very reticent to share potential mental health problems with others for fear of being stigmatised, particularly of being seen as 'crazy' by their friends. They don't want to need help, but want to sort things out for themselves and deal with their own issues. Young people are also unfamiliar with sources of potential help – this is not surprising, because they are at a time of life when most are physically healthy, and have no need for knowledge of health care providers. There are many structural, interpersonal and personal impediments to making use of the main sources of mental health care they have access to – the school counsellor and their family doctor.

Importantly, the very nature of the symptoms of the main mental health problems for young people actively works against seeking help. For example, depressive symptoms are associated with social withdrawal, meaning that young people pull away from rather than reach out to others. Depression is also characterised by lack of motivation and lethargy, which mitigate against taking action. Anxiety disorders are often social anxiety and generalised anxiety, which make young people embarrassed and fearful of seeking help from others – particularly strangers. Self-harm and the symptoms of eating disorders are perceived as shameful, needing to be hidden. Similarly, substance use must be concealed because it is illicit. If psychotic symptoms are present, loss of motivation and lack of touch with reality can severely compromise help-seeking behaviour. Suicide is probably the most frightening mental health issue for parents and significant others, and such thoughts are strongly associated with help-negation, which means actively *not* reaching out, particularly to parents. Most youth mental health issues are inherently associated with genuine fears about the consequences of disclosure and major barriers to seeking help.

WHO SHOULD REACH OUT?

Consequently, the caring adults in young people's lives have an important responsibility to reach out and intervene. They need to act in ways that overcome the many barriers to getting effective support for young people, and help them successfully deal with the mental health problems that are so common during the teen years.

There are many adults who are in regular contact with young people through their everyday lives and it is these people who know them best. They are the ones the young person knows and trusts, and who are in a position to notice problems, provide support and encourage seeking help. Parents are obviously the most important informal support for most young people, and research shows that teenagers generally turn to them first. This pattern is strongest early in adolescence and decreases with age, as expected with growing independence, but parents remain the primary informal support related to health and mental health issues throughout the teenage years. Although friends become an increasing source of support during adolescence, particularly for girls, parents remain primary.

Other adults can also play a significant role. In particular, close family members, teachers and coaches have frequent involvement with many young people and comprise important relationships in their lives. Young people respect and value the opinions of such adults, and their encouragement and advice can be very influential. For marginalised and at-risk young people, youth workers and counsellors can be critical supports. For young people with strong spiritual or religious beliefs, their spiritual advisors may be key connections. The significant caring adults in young people's lives need to recognise when young people are struggling with their mental health and know how to respond appropriately.

ROLE OF CARING ADULTS

Notice – what's going on for the young people you care about

Ask – reach out and ask them how they are

Know – what resources are available online and in your local area

WHAT ARE THE SIGNS FOR CONCERN?

Knowing when to really be concerned and when not to is important. Adolescence is a time of such significant change that it's hard to know what's 'normal' and to be expected, and what's not. There are many major changes happening at this time of life – physically, socially, emotionally and cognitively. Young people and their families cope with these in diverse ways that depend on gender, the timing of puberty, culture, family make-up, local environment, sexual orientation, and many other factors. But, just because something is widespread among youth doesn't mean it is 'normal' and has to be accepted as an inevitable part of adolescence.

The main thing in knowing whether to be concerned or not is to trust your own feelings, and get informed. Trusted adults are in a unique position with a young person they know well. They will notice when something is not quite right.

Things you might notice that are cause for concern include:

- Self-harm – any indicator of this (cuts, burns) is a warning sign that something is wrong.
- Sleep problems – changes in sleep patterns are typical in adolescence, but ongoing major sleep disturbance is a concern. Eliminating any reasons for poor sleep is the first step, but if this doesn't help, get professional support. Good sleep is essential for teenage wellbeing.
- Social withdrawal – spending time secluded in their (often very messy) bedroom is a teenage stereotype, and the (unfortunately common) practice of allowing technological devices in bedrooms encourages this. The more a young person withdraws socially from family, and from friends, the greater the cause for concern.
- Losing interest in usual activities – during adolescence many young people give up on the activities they were very engaged with during childhood. This can be attributed to changing identity and friendship groups, but losing interest

in key pleasurable activities like arts, sports and music can be a sign.

- Disordered eating – unhealthy eating behaviours are all too common, especially for girls, and these are encouraged and reinforced by modern media. But changes in a young person's relationship with food, such as constant dieting or restricted eating behaviours, are a reason to worry.
- Bullying, cyberbullying – we now know that experience of bullying is a serious risk factor for young people's mental health and wellbeing, and young people require strong support to effectively deal with bullying behaviours.
- Relationship problems – these are another major risk factor, particularly family breakdown and family violence.
- Engaging in risky behaviours – engaging in early sexual activity and substance use are risks in and of themselves, but often are also indicators of other problems.
- Poor body image – teenage girls are stereotyped for excessive grooming and concern about their appearance, but poor body image and excessive body dissatisfaction in both girls and boys can become a serious mental health issue.
- Lack of self-care – teenage boys tend to be stereotyped as not caring much about their appearance or cleanliness, but ongoing self-care issues can be cause for concern.

IT *IS* OKAY TO ASK

The list provided above is not exhaustive, but shows some of the indicators for concern that might be noticed by those close to and in regular contact with young people. Many other mental health problems are not easily observable, however, and the only way to find out what is going on with a young person is to ask.

One very simple technique for checking how a young person is faring is to ask them how they are currently feeling on a scale from 0 to 10, with 0 being the worst possible and 10 being the best possible. This is an easy and non-intrusive way to regularly check in. To first introduce this technique, pick a good time, when everything is calm, and explain the nature of the scale. Then, a simple 'Hey, where are you on 0 to 10 at the moment?' provides a way to quickly check in whenever needed. While each young person is different, responses between 6 and 9 usually mean that things are likely to be okay. Below 6 indicates that things might be getting off track. At the other end of the scale, being a 10 too often without good reason might be cause for concern.

On the more serious side of checking in, one of the main myths related to mental health is that asking about suicide puts thoughts of it into a young person's head. We now know that this is not true. Talking about suicide does not make it happen, although it is important to be careful not to normalise suicide as a coping strategy, nor to dwell on celebrity suicides or the means by which people have suicided. But if you are concerned that a young person may be at risk of suicide, you can ask them questions such as: *Do you feel like giving up? Are you thinking about hurting yourself? Do you think living is not worthwhile? Do you feel like you'd be better off dead?* If they reveal that they are thinking this way, go on to ask them if they have a plan for how and when they would harm themselves. If they have any sort of plan, take it seriously – stay with them, remove any obvious means if possible, and get professional help. Suicidal ideation should always be taken seriously.

CONVERSATIONS AND COMMUNICATION

When talking to young people about their mental health it is essential to be non-judgemental – young people are extraordinarily attuned to detecting judgement, disapproval and criticism. Be open and accepting of everything they say. Listen carefully and unconditionally. Ask open-ended questions and reflect back what they say to show you are truly listening. Take care to ensure that your facial expressions and body language also convey acceptance and tolerance. This can be hard, especially if you are a parent who is very worried about what is being disclosed. Note that this does not mean acting like their best friend. Being non-judgemental is not about condoning risky behaviour; rather, it means listening as a respectful, compassionate and responsible adult who is in control of themselves and their reactions, and has the young person's wellbeing as their utmost concern.

The aim of such conversations is to find out what is going on for the young person, validate their feelings, have them feel supported and safe, determine their level of risk, and help them access further help if required. The goal is not to figure out and solve their problems. Nor is it to minimise or dismiss their feelings and concerns. Take what they say seriously. Teenage feelings are more intense, immediate and distressing than those experienced by most adults about similar concerns; adults have much more life experience to draw upon. Adolescents haven't had the chance to develop a longer-term perspective and tend to get more highly distressed.

If you are trying to encourage a young person to take a particular health action, note that they are not generally motivated by consequences, particularly scare tactics. The executive function parts of the brain are the last to mature – this doesn't happen until well into the twenties – so rationalisation often doesn't work for teens, especially when they are highly distressed or aroused. Their brains are still functioning largely through the more primitive emotional arousal systems, rather than via the brain systems controlling reason and planning, so appealing to their emotions and need to reduce immediate distress is more helpful.

Adolescents are also uniquely attuned to their peers, so referencing other young people their age can encourage action. It is very helpful for young people to know that they are not alone in their mental health-related experiences, and that they are not going to be socially penalised for what they are going through. Peers are an increasingly important social reference point, and acceptance by peers is critical, with maximal impact around mid-adolescence. Peers can be both a source of encouragement and support, and also a reason for significant concerns about stigma, confidentiality and social exclusion due to being different and not fitting in.

USING SOCIAL REFERENCING TO ENCOURAGE SEEKING HELP

'You seem to be pretty down. How are you feeling? … Young people your age often feel pretty down – there's a lot going on … Are you going through a tough time? What's happening for you? … There are some things many people your age find really helpful. One is checking out some of the info available online. Lots of young people say that this has been really useful for them. The content is often developed by young people themselves – to help each other out. How would you feel about checking out some info online at a website specifically designed for young people feeling like you do?'

THE FIRST STEP IS ONLINE

One of the first steps in moving beyond informal support to seeking professional help is through the use of online resources. The development of online support specifically for young people is growing and there are a number of excellent youth-specific websites available. These provide relevant information for young people as well as those who care for them.

Technology has emerged as a critical gateway for youth mental health as its use is embedded in young people's lives. It has huge potential to break down barriers to accessing mental health support and is increasingly seen as the most appropriate first step. The value of technology and the online environment is that it is easy, free, can be available anytime and anywhere, can be entirely private, the young person feels in control, and it's non-stigmatising. The rapidly expanding range of online and technology-enabled interventions makes them vital links in the help-seeking process.

Importantly, online interventions provide a 'soft-entry' point where young people can try out some aspects of mental health support. Easy access to psycho-education and self-help screening tools can help young people, and the adults who care for them, identify mental health needs and appropriate actions to take. Interestingly, many young people say they find it 'easier to type than talk' about personally sensitive issues.

Technology has a role across the whole spectrum of support, from mental health promotion, prevention and early intervention, through to continuing care and recovery for those who develop longer-term conditions.

All young people need support for their mental health and wellbeing. Online resources are a great place for encouraging development of good life habits for all young people (and not so young people!). This includes sleep hygiene, the importance of sunlight and vitamin D, how to eat well, techniques to regularly de-stress (e.g. meditation, physical activity), and learning basic cognitive and behavioural skills to be 'mentally fit' to deal with distressing thoughts and feelings (e.g. mindfulness).

Many websites facilitate communication from and between young people, and support online communities where young people can find support from peers. This peer connection and sense of belonging can be critical for young people experiencing mental health problems and related risk factors, and young people are often more likely to take actions supported by a peer (rather than a parent). However, it is essential that young people are guided to online and technological resources that are evidence based and appropriately moderated.

YOUTH-SPECIFIC WEBSITES

YoungMinds: youngminds.org.uk

Mind: www.mind.org.uk

CALM (Campaign, Against Living Miserably – for men): www.thecalmzone.net

PAPYRUS (prevention of young suicide): www.papyrus-uk.org

SupportLine: www.supportline.org.uk

Youth Access: www.youthaccess.org.uk/supernav/links

The Mix: www.themix.org.uk

NEXT STEPS

One problem with online and 'self-help' options is that young people can find it hard to engage with them, and either drop off pretty quickly or won't try them out at all. This is a particular challenge for those who lack motivation, feel lethargic and hopeless, and think that nothing will help. In this case, professionals who are skilled in working with young people need to become involved. Sometimes their role can be to support and guide the young person through the resources that are available online and via technology. This 'guided self-help' is increasingly understood to be one of the most effective approaches. Providing the professionals who work regularly with young people, like teachers and youth workers, with such skills will greatly improve access to support, and unlock the huge potential of the growing array of evidence-based online resources.

Face-to-face services are often required, however, particularly when issues are acute or complex, or the young person won't engage in other support. The people who care for and work with young people need to know which appropriate services are available in their local area. Often the school counsellor, school psychologist or youth worker is a good first option, although such services are not always available or appropriate. The family doctor is another possibility, although some young people become reluctant to see them with sensitive, personal problems. If your area has a youth-specific medical, counselling or mental health service, these are specifically designed to be engaging and appropriate for youth. Accredited psychologists can be found through the Find a Psychologist service of the British Psychological Society (www.bps.org.uk).

More serious mental ill health will require additional specialist intervention, such as psychiatry. Your general practitioner, psychologist, or youth health service will know how to refer.

DON'T GIVE UP

Unfortunately, young people can remain reluctant to seek help; and sometimes, after considerable effort to get a young person to access services, the source of help does not provide a good experience or is simply not the right fit. This is distressing for all involved, as the window of opportunity to get a young person to accept help can be small and close quickly. Here is where our service system and its providers need to step up and ensure that engaging, non-judgemental, non-stigmatising, appropriate and effective service responses are widely available to all young people when they are ready to seek help.

But don't give up. Wait for another time. It is the nature of mental health issues, and their associated distress, that they tend to come and go. This means there will be another opportunity. Keep checking in with your young person. Become better informed and more prepared for the next time – more confident in how to communicate with them and ready with knowledge of the best directions in which to point them. Research shows that parents and caring adults need to persevere in their efforts to find young people with emerging mental ill health the support they need.

LAST WORD

Look after yourself. Research shows that the mental wellbeing of the parents and carers of young people with mental health problems is significantly at risk. This is partly due to 'activity restriction', which means curtailing social, occupational and personal activities because of the impact of their young person's mental health problems. It is essential to look after yourself, maintain your own social connections and meaningful activities. We all need to take care of ourselves, and look after our own mental wellbeing, before we can effectively help others.

Author biography

Dr Debra Rickwood is Professor of Psychology at the University of Canberra and Chief Scientific Officer for headspace, Australia's National Youth Mental Health Foundation. She is a Fellow of the Australian Psychological Society and has researched extensively the factors that affect young people seeking help for mental health problems.

www.headspace.org.au

See also:
Chapter 2: What to do in a Mental Health Crisis

Recommended websites:
Mind: www.mind.org.uk
Royal College of Psychiatrists: www.rcpsych.ac.uk/healthadivce
Mental Health Foundation: www.mentalhealth.org.uk

Further reading:

Carr-Gregg, M 2010, *When to Really Worry*, Penguin Books Australia, Camberwell.

Centre of Excellence in Youth Mental Health 2010, *MythBuster: Sorting Fact from Fiction on Self-Harm*, Orygen Youth Health Research Centre, Melbourne.

Centre of Excellence in Youth Mental Health 2009, *MythBuster: Suicidal Ideation*, Orygen Youth Health Research Centre, Melbourne.

Rickwood, DJ 2014, 'Responding effectively to support the mental health and well-being of young people', in Cahill, H & Wyn, J (Eds.), *Handbook of Children and Youth Studies*, Springer, USA, pp 139–154.

2. WHAT TO DO IN A MENTAL HEALTH CRISIS

Dr Claire Kelly

Mental illness is common in young people. To encourage them to seek and accept help, adults can learn simple mental health first aid skills and communication techniques. This chapter is written for teachers in particular.

INTRODUCTION

Mental illness is common in young people, and carries with it a high degree of disability. Young people often do not seek the help they need, because of embarrassment, shyness or a fear of negative judgement. However, most mental illnesses can be effectively treated, and seeking help early can prevent mental illness from becoming severe and long lasting. Mental health first aid skills, in combination with communication techniques that facilitate open conversation, can enable adults to encourage young people to seek and accept help. These skills are not difficult to learn.

WHAT IS MENTAL HEALTH FIRST AID?

Mental health first aid is the help given to a person who is developing a mental health problem, experiencing a worsening of a mental health problem, or in a mental health crisis. Mental health first aid is provided until help has been received, or the crisis has resolved.

This chapter will describe the development of the Mental Health First Aid programme, and take readers through an example of using the skills taught in the programme to assist a young person with a mental health problem.

Mental Health First Aid was first conceived in 2000 by Ms Betty Kitchener and Professor Tony Jorm. Ms Kitchener had a broad range of professional and life experiences. She had been a nurse and a first aid instructor, and a person who had struggled with severe depression at various times in her life. Professor Jorm, her husband, was a highly regarded researcher in psychology and mental health. They discussed the possibility of a first aid course that would teach members of the public to help a friend, family member, colleague or other member of the public who was beginning to show signs of mental health problems. The focus would be similar to the focus in first aid: facilitating early intervention.

One of the drivers for this work was the 1997 Australian National Survey of Mental Health Literacy. Mental health literacy is defined as 'knowledge and beliefs about mental disorders which aid their recognition, management or prevention. Mental health literacy includes the ability to recognise specific disorders; knowing how to seek mental health information; knowledge of risk factors and causes, of self-treatments, and of professional help available; and attitudes that promote recognition and appropriate help-seeking.'[1] This study showed that Australians had poor understanding of mental illness, were not readily able to identify depression or a developing psychotic disorder, and had poor knowledge of treatments appropriate for treating mental illnesses. The study also revealed a high level of stigma in the Australian community and attitudes that were not conducive to treatment-seeking.

In the early 2000s, the Mental Health First Aid programme began locally in Canberra, Australia. It expanded across Australia in the next few years, and began to travel overseas in 2003, when it was adopted by the Scottish government. It has since spread to over twenty countries. As of January 2017, over two million people had completed the training worldwide.

Research on Mental Health First Aid training has been conducted in Australia and several other countries, including uncontrolled trials, randomised controlled trials and qualitative research. A meta-analysis of the results of the randomised controlled trials was conducted by Swedish researchers in 2013. It was found that Mental Health First Aid training improves recognition of mental illnesses, increases congruence with professional beliefs about treatments, and decreases stigmatising attitudes. Mental Health First Aid training decreases stigma as much as programmes designed with stigma reduction as their primary aim.[2]

Mental health first aid skills

Mental Health First Aid Australia teaches mental health first aid skills based on a series of guidelines developed with the assistance of hundreds of experts across English-speaking countries with comparable health systems. The Delphi method enables researchers to build and reach consensus in large groups. The mental health first aid guidelines draw on a broad range of experiences and different kinds of expertise, by engaging panels of mental health professionals (clinical experts and researchers), and people with lived experience of mental illness (either personal experience, or as a significant caregiver such as a parent, spouse or close friend).

Mental health first aid guidelines have been developed for a range of mental illnesses and crisis situations. Mental illnesses covered include depression, psychosis, eating disorders, alcohol use problems, other substance use problems, gambling and confusion (generally confusion related to dementia). Crisis situations include suicidal thoughts and behaviours, non-suicidal self-injury, traumatic events and panic attacks. There is a range of crisis situations covered by the guidelines for specific mental illnesses as well, such as assisting in a medical emergency related to substance use or eating disorders, assisting when someone is becoming aggressive, and assisting with severe psychosis.

There are additional guidelines to help apply mental health first aid to particular groups. For example, there are guidelines to assist adults to talk with young people about mental illness and other sensitive or difficult topics, guidelines to assist in discussing mental illness with young Aboriginal and Torres Strait Islander people, and guidelines on providing mental health first aid sensitively to a lesbian, gay, bisexual, transgender, intersex, queer or questioning (LGBTIQ) person. Guidelines for some specific professional groups and more specialised settings are also available from the Mental Health First Aid website.

Mental health first aid and young people

While everyone can benefit from mental health first aid skills, it is especially important that people who work with and care for young people have these skills. Adolescence is the peak age of onset for mental illness, and half of all people who will ever have a mental illness will have their first episode before they are eighteen years old.[3] Young people often lack insight and are less likely than adults to identify they have a problem that will benefit from professional help. They usually lack psychological maturity and life experience that would prompt them to actively seek help for themselves. Young people are unlikely to seek help unless an adult they trust encourages them to or facilitates the help-seeking directly.

Adults in the community – family members, teachers, community leaders, coaches, tutors, employers and others – need the knowledge (or 'mental health literacy') and skills to apply mental health first aid.

Similar to a traditional first aid course, mental health first aid is not designed to teach a member of the public to diagnose a mental illness or provide treatment of any kind.

THE MENTAL HEALTH OF YOUNG PEOPLE

Mental illness is common in adolescents. Recent research in Australia found that based on the report of their parents, 14 per cent of twelve- to seventeen-year-olds have some form of mental illness in a twelve-month period.[4] This figure is conservative, as the research covered only a limited range of illnesses, and young people reporting on their own mental health cite more symptoms. Among young adults the figure is even higher, with more than a quarter meeting criteria for a mental illness in the last twelve months.[5]

Assisting young people to seek help early can decrease the impact that mental illness can have on development and educational outcomes, set up better help-seeking habits for life, and may decrease the likelihood of later episodes.

USING MENTAL HEALTH FIRST AID SKILLS TO HELP A YOUNG PERSON

Although every situation is different, the mental health first aid guidelines can be used and adapted to help most people in most situations. In addition, they offer guidance on what to do if the young person is resistant to help.

In this chapter, we will apply mental health first aid skills to help a young woman, Jessica, who is displaying signs of a developing mental health problem. The advice in this chapter will draw mainly from *Communicating with adolescents: guidelines for adults on how to communicate with adolescents about mental health problems and other sensitive topics*[6] and *Depression: first aid guidelines.*[7]

Meet Jessica

Jessica is a student in your class who recently turned seventeen. When she was younger she was sometimes described as a difficult child, often argumentative with adults and resistant to attending school. She is intelligent and when she applies herself she does well, though she has never been willing to work hard on anything she is not interested in. Jessica has only a small number of close friends, and resists doing anything that will bring her into contact with anyone new.

Six months ago, Jessica's parents separated. You are aware that there had been a great deal of fighting in the months before Jessica's father moved out. Jessica has mentioned in class that she gets along better with her father than her mother. She and her mother have been fighting since he left, and she doesn't see a lot of her father. She is angry with her mother about the separation. The anger is spilling out elsewhere; she appears to be in conflict with her friends at least once or twice a week.

You are concerned that her performance in your class, which she has described as one of her favourites, has taken a very sharp decline in the last two weeks.

There is nothing in the story so far that indicates that Jessica has significant mental health problems. It is quite normal for a young person to be upset and angry during a major upheaval.

However, Jessica has a number of risk factors for the development of a mental health problem. Having been described as 'difficult' when she was young could mean a range of different things. She is reticent in social situations, so she may have had a school phobia or social phobia; half of all people who will ever have an anxiety disorder have had their first episode before the age of fifteen. The recent separation is also a risk factor, particularly as it seems to have had a great impact on her. Adolescence is the peak age of onset, and more females than males develop mental illness.

Risk factors are useful to be aware of because they can guide prevention efforts. They can also help to alert adults to monitor young people who are more vulnerable to developing problems. However, risk factors cannot tell us who has a mental health problem and, as such, are not as helpful to helpers as an awareness of the symptoms of mental health problems.

Initially, you are going to speak to Jessica as her teacher. However, it's useful to take into consideration her vulnerability. Using the guidelines for communicating about sensitive topics, there are a few things worth keeping in mind.

Preparing your approach

At this stage, you don't know what the focus of your conversation with Jessica is likely to be. It is safe to assume that it's going to be a difficult conversation for her and possibly for you as well. If she feels attacked, it will be hard to have a productive conversation, so it's good to keep a few things in mind to reduce the chances of her becoming defensive.

The approach you take with Jessica is very important. It can be very confronting to ask her to stay, in front of the entire class. Approach her where neither of you are likely to be the centre of attention and ask if she has time to talk. If not, arrange a time to do so. This needs to be at a time and a place where your focus won't be divided and no one is likely to interrupt.

What to say

It is important to talk to Jessica as a concerned person, and not as an 'expert' or superior. Allow her to control the conversation, as far as possible, while making sure you find the space to express your concerns. Allow plenty of time for silence as she may need time to process what you're saying. Be ready to steer the conversation in the direction of mental health or distress if needed.

Let her know that you care and want to help, and ask if she wants to talk about anything. If she doesn't, point out the specific things you have noticed and explain why you are concerned.

You arrange a time to speak to Jessica, later in the afternoon. You let her know she's not in trouble, but you are concerned about the changes in her performance in class. You tell her that you're aware that her family has experienced a tough time lately and you would like to offer her some support to avoid her grades dropping any further. She is uncommunicative initially, shrugging and refusing to make eye contact, with her arms crossed over her chest. However, she starts to appear visibly distressed, and looks like she might be trying to stop herself from crying. She tells you quite aggressively that she isn't sleeping properly and she's tired, and that's all there is to it. When you suggest she should perhaps consider going to bed earlier, she says she sometimes lies in bed feeling sick or with a headache.

When you ask if there is anything else bothering her, she says no. She tells you she'll work harder, and asks if she can leave.

WHAT SIGNS SHOULD I BE LOOKING FOR?

The common mental illnesses among adolescents are depression and anxiety disorders. It's useful to be aware of some of the symptoms of these illnesses. You can easily find lists of symptoms on the internet, or elsewhere in this book. It is important to read and consider these, as some of the symptoms can easily be mistaken for normal adolescent mood changes. There are many different anxiety disorders with a wide range of symptoms that can appear disrespectful (avoidance of situations, ignoring people because of social anxiety) or even antisocial (such as being quick to lose temper), and having an understanding that such behaviour might be a sign of anxiety can make it easier to avoid being confrontational.

Although it's good to have a basic understanding of these symptoms, this simple definition of mental illness can provide guidance about when to act.

A mental health problem is:

1. Major changes in thoughts, feelings or behaviour
2. . . . that interfere with functioning
3. . . . and don't go away quickly.

The specific symptoms don't matter as much as the severity, impact and duration.

By now, you've observed some symptoms that are of concern, and you want to talk to Jessica about the possibility of a mental health problem and suggest she seeks some help.

You are not trying to make a diagnosis of any specific illness, just trying to determine whether she needs some help. Read the box titled 'What signs should I be looking for?' Consider how that guidance fits with what we have seen of Jessica so far.

Some of the symptoms you are now aware of are:

- She is no longer enjoying things she used to enjoy.
- There is interpersonal conflict.
- She is having difficulty sleeping.
- She feels sick and is having headaches.
- She is weepy.

These symptoms are interfering with Jessica's ability to get by day to day, as evidenced by the decline in her grades and her fighting with her friends. The changes have been especially pronounced over the last two weeks. This means that you are not observing the occasional bad day; you are making note of a significant change.

It's important to note as well that after any major life event, such as parental separation, there is bound to be a period of associated upset or distress. In Jessica's case, this distress has carried on for six months, with a sudden worsening. Dismissing what you have noticed as normal is not helpful. As with any distressing life event, if things don't improve, this can signal the onset of mental health problems.

Handling difficulties in the conversation

Jessica is reluctant to talk, but you need to do something. A reluctance to talk to you right now is not the same as a refusal to do anything at all. Reiterate that you care about Jessica, and want to help. Consider your body language and make sure you are not towering over her or doing anything that might make you look angry.

Let her know she doesn't have to reveal anything to you that she doesn't want to or is not ready to. You are not going to try to provide any therapy. Emphasise that help is available, and you can facilitate her getting the help that she needs.

It might be that you are not the right person to talk to her about what is happening. You could ask her if there is someone else at the school who she is willing to talk to about how she's feeling. A school psychologist or school counsellor might be less intimidating if she is feeling upset about her grades. Or it might be that she would prefer to speak to someone of a different age or gender. Try not to take it personally. Instead, discuss options for who you could help her talk to.

ASSESSING FOR SUICIDAL THOUGHTS

There is nothing immediately apparent that suggests that Jessica is having thoughts of suicide. However, as she open up, you need to listen carefully for:

- Expressions of helplessness and hopelessness: 'There's no point; everything sucks, and nothing is ever going to change.'
- Talking about being a burden: 'Everyone would be better off without me.'
- Talk of death and dying, or wishing to be dead: 'Sometimes I wish I could just go to sleep and never wake up.'

The risk of suicide should never be taken lightly. The chapter in this book titled 'Suicide and Attempted Suicide' can guide you to assisting a young person who is having thoughts of suicide.

She may also just need more time. Do not presume she doesn't want your help. Adolescents may struggle to ask for help or accept help that has been offered to them, even if they don't feel they have control over the situation they are in, and are motivated to seek a change. If you have seen no sign that Jessica may be in crisis, or at immediate risk, you could let her leave and tell her you're going to follow up with her in a day or two to see how things are going.

With some time to consider what you've said, she might be in a better space to discuss what has been happening and how she is feeling. This means that it is really important that when you've said you will follow up, you do so. It's important to be as consistent and reliable as you can.

As Jessica does not appear to be in immediate danger, you tell her that you'd like to talk to her again tomorrow, and ask her to meet you at lunchtime. She is there on time, and although she does not immediately appear to want to talk, she seems more relaxed and makes eye contact. You ask her if she's thought about the things the two of you discussed and she says she has.

She admits that it's been more difficult than she has been letting on. Sometimes she can't stop crying and at other times she feels angry with everyone, particularly her mother. She hasn't had much of an appetite and she's lost weight, because she so often feels sick. Everything seems to be getting more difficult over time. She can't enjoy anything, and everything seems hopeless.

Jessica has begun to open up to you, and you're probably hearing more than you were anticipating. On top of the symptoms you were aware of, you've now learned that things are getting worse, that her tearfulness and poor temper are a chronic problem, and that she has had an appetite change that has led to weight loss.

Providing information

You've seen some signs of depression and anxiety. You are not going to make any kind of diagnosis, but it's fine to acknowledge that you've seen a cluster of symptoms that suggest that Jessica is struggling with depression and anxiety.

If Jessica is willing, you could go online together and look at some good-quality websites. Many have screening questionnaires. Jessica could complete one of these to get a sense of how her moods compare to others', and this may help her make a decision to seek help. Many of these websites have fact sheets. If Jessica is reluctant to continue the conversation right now, she might be willing to take some reading material away with her. Don't be forceful about this. It can take a few mental health first aid conversations before the young person agrees to talk to someone who can provide some kind of treatment. Unless the young person is in crisis, it's okay to take your time. It is better to have the young person committed to seeking help and guiding this themselves to the greatest degree possible rather than try to force them to accept help and have them refuse to engage.

ADVICE FOR PARENTS

It can be frustrating and upsetting to try to assist your own child when they appear reluctant to talk to you, or reluctant to accept professional help. It can feel like rejection, and is often difficult not to take personally. Here are some tips that can help you make progress when it seems like you're both stuck:

- Ask if there is someone else your child would feel more willing to talk to. A member of your extended family, a family friend, or another adult your child is close to might be able to help.
- Unless there is imminent risk of harm, give it a day or two and try again. Remember that mental health problems don't arise quickly, and they don't go away quickly either.
- Providing consistent emotional support and remaining calm and ready to talk when they feel able to can make it easier for them to come back to you when they've considered what you have said.

Seek appropriate professional help

Jessica's difficulties have been persistent over time and a sudden worsening will have you worried. It's important that Jessica has an assessment from a mental health professional.

> You suggest to Jessica that it would be a good idea to talk to someone who can help her understand what is happening. Jessica says that all she needs is someone to talk to, and she's willing to talk to you, but no one else.
>
> However, her symptoms warrant professional assessment, and possibly treatment. She reiterates that she doesn't need 'that kind of help', and refuses once more.

It's important that you keep the relationship positive, but you don't want to enable her to avoid getting help. You're quite concerned. Without suggesting that you won't have any part of it, you want to make sure that she understands just how seriously you are taking this. There are some things you can try saying that might encourage her, such as:

-

- 'You and I can still talk, but I'm really concerned about how upset you've been lately. I don't have the right kind of training to help you if this is a mental health problem. Let's talk with someone who can at least figure out what kind of help you might need.'
- 'You might be right – maybe you just need some extra support, and I'm willing to give you that. But it might be that support won't be enough. A mental health professional can work out what you might need, and they might be able to give me some advice about how I can support you better.'
- 'A lot of the time, people are reluctant to seek help because they have an idea of what treatment might involve and they don't like it. Can you tell me what you think might happen if you talk to a mental health professional?'

You decide to find out what is behind Jessica's reluctance.

Jessica admits that she saw a film once where a girl was depressed, and took medication that made her feel like a zombie. She also spent several weeks in hospital, where she was forced to talk about her childhood. Jessica thinks she might have the same kind of problem. She doesn't want to take medication, she doesn't want to go to hospital, and she had a happy childhood.

You explain to Jessica that movies often promote stereotypes that are inaccurate. The most effective treatment for most mental health problems is talk therapy. The most common kind is Cognitive Behavioural Therapy (CBT), which helps people to understand that the way they think affects the way they feel, which in turn affects the way they behave. It's practical, and it focuses on working to change the way you think, rather than trying to figure out why things began to go wrong. For example, CBT might help her to think differently about her parents' separation, and the conflict with her friends.

Jessica agrees to talk to someone just once to find out what it is all about.

There are a number of different professionals who can help.

You could suggest that she talks to her GP. You could offer to talk to her mother or to be present while she talks to her mother, to discuss getting an appointment.

If there is a youth-focused mental health or health service close by, you could help her to arrange to see someone there.

As you are in a school setting, the school counsellor might be a good option. You have some momentum with Jessica now and it would be good to keep it going and seek help now or today.

Jessica agrees to talk to the school counsellor, just to find out what they think about what's happening, and only if you go along. Once they begin to talk, Jessica feels more able to agree to speak to the counsellor alone.

Your role as a mental health first aider ends when Jessica begins talking to the school counsellor. You may continue to offer support, however, and you will follow school policies on how to make reasonable adjustments to allow Jessica to begin pulling her grades up, e.g. allowing extra time on homework and exams. The counsellor will take responsibility for assisting Jessica with her mental health, including making a recommendation for further referral if needed, and ideally getting Jessica's parents involved.

CONCLUSION

Helping a young person who is struggling with mental illness can be challenging. However, simple mental health first aid skills, and guidance around communicating effectively with young people, can help. If a young person believes that an adult genuinely cares about them and wants to help, they are more likely to accept help that has been offered. Patience and persistence are important keys to this process. Unless a young person is in crisis, it's okay to take a little while to get them to accept help. Being a consistent support through this process and beyond can help them to achieve a good recovery.

Author biography

Dr Claire Kelly is the manager of youth programmes at Mental Health First Aid Australia. She has been a main contributor to the mental health first aid guidelines projects. Claire has experienced episodes of depression and anxiety since early adolescence, which has been a driver for her work.

www.mhfa.com.au

See also:
Chapter 1: Helping Young People Get Help for Mental Health Problems
Chapter 22: Understanding the Teenage Brain

Recommended website:
Mental Health First Aid: www.mhfaengland.org

Further reading:
Kelly, CM, Kitchener, BA & Jorm, AF 2017, *Youth Mental Health First Aid: A Manual for Adults Assisting Young People* (4th ed), Mental Health First Aid Australia, Melbourne.
Purcell R, Ryan S, Scanlan F, Morgan A, Callahan P, Allen N & Jorm A 2013, *A Guide to What Works for Depression in Young People* (2nd ed), beyondblue, Melbourne.

 For more online resources visit:
generationnext.com.au/handbook

COMMON MENTAL HEALTH CONCERNS

Bullying Basics   35

Anxiety in Young People   53

Depression in Young People   64

Understanding Self-harm   80

Suicide and Attempted Suicide   96

Towards Prevention: Understanding Child Sexual Assault   114

3. BULLYING BASICS

Sandra Craig

This chapter is about bullying – what it is, what it isn't, what to do and not do about it – for parents, teachers and others working with young people.

INTRODUCTION

Most of us know – or think we know – what bullying is. Many have experienced bullying at school, sporting clubs or in the workplace. A similar number, at some time or other, will have been involved in bullying others. There are many reasons for both of these patterns. Some will carry scars from those events for much of their lives, but not all. This chapter will try to show some of the subtleties, complexities and nuances connected to bullying. However, because bullying takes place in social situations and involves interactions between personalities, it's impossible to cover every type of bullying situation.

When I was a teacher, enraged parents frequently accosted me during the day demanding I did something about the bullying their child was experiencing. Often it took a considerable while to get to the core of what had happened. And often it wasn't bullying at all.

When I began in my role as manager of the National Centre Against Bullying (NCAB) in Australia, I thought it possible to construct a standard reply to all queries from parents, teachers and others, but quickly had to discard that idea. Each situation was very different and so for the last nine years, every reply has been a response to a unique set of circumstances.

BULLYING MATTERS

Awareness of the level and impact of bullying in society has generated a rising concern in many parts of the world about its prevalence, seriousness and negative effects and has encouraged schools, workplaces and other environments to address it seriously.

We now recognise bullying as a human rights issue.

A recent (2016) NCAB conference presented clear evidence of the psychological and traumatic impact of bullying and its long-term impact on the health and wellbeing of people who have been consistently bullied and of persistent bullies.

There is a range of problematic effects of bullying which can persist over the course of someone's life. For the child or young person who bullies and does not receive support to stop the behaviour, these can include:

- anger and misconduct
- growing up without a clear understanding of the difference between right and wrong
- criminal or delinquent behaviour later in life (e.g. workplace bullying, assault, theft, sexual harassment, domestic violence).

For the target of bullying, these can include:

- poor physical health
- low self-esteem
- depression
- anxiety disorders
- school avoidance
- deterioration in school work.

There are many school-based programmes designed to prevent bullying, but few programmes specifically target the behaviour of bystanders (i.e. someone who witnesses bullying). However, bystanders are nearly always present when bullying happens – up to 80 per cent of the time. These bystanders play different roles but very often do not intervene on behalf of the target of bullying. The bullying incidents can have lasting negative effects on these young people who, like it or not, are implicated in the events they observe.

Young people who intervene in bullying incidents can reduce victimisation by around 50 per cent. But it's important that this happens in an environment supportive of bystander intervention and where students are effectively trained. Bystanders can intervene by:

- Reporting the incident.
- Supporting the student who is being targeted.
- Directly intervening when it is safe – that is, the bystander is confident the bullying will not be turned on them.

We are used to horror stories in the media, but it's important to bear in mind that, even though the numbers of bullied children and young people remain unacceptably high, there is not 'an epidemic' of bullying. The good news is that the work that schools are doing to address bullying is having an impact. Two large-scale, robust Australian studies, conducted seven years apart, show a reduction from 27 per cent of students bullied to 19.8 per cent.

BULLYING – DEFINED (SORT OF)

So what is bullying? Different commentators define it in slightly different ways, but there is general agreement that bullying is an ongoing misuse of power in relationships through repeated aggressive verbal, physical and/or social behaviour on or offline, which intends to cause physical and/or psychological harm, distress or fear. It can involve an individual or a group misusing their power over one or more persons. Bullying can happen in person or online, and it can be obvious (overt) or hidden (covert). It always happens in social environments, whether online or offline.

We have often seen bullying as a predicament for an individual – i.e. the bullied person. However, as we will show, bullying also creates problems for those who bully, those who witness the bullying and others who are threatened merely by the fact of bullying taking place in their environment.

Bullying can occur at almost any time in a person's life. Several researchers have suggested that bullying by peers emerges when children start to interact socially and they have identified that preschool children also participate in direct and indirect bullying, including verbal bullying, social exclusion and rumour spreading. Bullying tends to increase when young people encounter others in a new social environment, such as when students enter secondary school.

Examples of bullying include:

- Verbal or written abuse – such as targeted name-calling or jokes, or displaying offensive posters.
- Violence – including threats of violence.
- Hostile behaviour towards students in relation to gender and sexuality.
- Telling stories about people known to be untrue in order to turn others against them.
- Discrimination and exclusion including racial discrimination – treating people differently because of their identity.
- Cyberbullying – either online or via mobile phone.

Bullying does not include:

- Mutual conflict that involves disagreement, but not an imbalance of power; unresolved mutual conflict can develop into bullying if one of the parties targets the other repeatedly in retaliation.
- Single-episode acts of nastiness or physical aggression, or aggression directed towards many different people.
- Social rejection or dislike unless it involves deliberate and repeated attempts to cause distress, exclude, or create dislike by others.

How should we talk about bullying?

- It's important to use language that doesn't label either participant in a bullying incident, as young people are rarely engaged in bullying continually or, for that matter, bullied for their whole lives. Labels have a way of sticking and can cause unfair judgements about that young person.
- So, rather than 'bully', NCAB uses terms such as 'bullying student' or 'person doing the bullying' even though it is more clumsily worded. Rather than using 'victim', which further disempowers the other student, we suggest using the term 'target'.
- This terminology also reflects the fact that roles in bullying situations are frequently fluid and a target can become a perpetrator and vice versa.

Where does bullying happen?

- Bullying tends to take place when adults are not around. This includes the corridors, locker areas, canteen and playground, behind buildings and in classrooms when a teacher is late or has left the room. Supervision is essential but full supervision of all areas where students congregate is just not possible.

How can I tell if it's bullying?

Young children will tell adults what is bothering them, but as they become teenagers they are less likely to tell parents/carers or teachers that they are being bullied; and boys are much less apt to disclose than are girls. In fact, bullied children are more likely to tell friends than their teachers.

Sometimes the only thing parents and teachers can do is to be on the alert for changes in behaviour that can indicate that something might be wrong at school, sporting club or other social venue.

Things for parents to watch for at home

Parents or carers might notice changes of mood that show up in unexplained anger or tears, or changes in behaviour such as sleep patterns, nightmares, bedwetting and withdrawal from family, social groups or friends. A young person might be unwilling to go to school or will come home hungry, or with unexplained scratches, bruises, or lost, torn or broken belongings. They might lose or gain weight suddenly. They might wear long-sleeved clothing even in summer as a means of hiding extreme weight loss or evidence of self-harm. They may offer unconvincing explanations for any of these.

Things for teachers to watch for at school

A young person might talk of wanting to leave school, might be in trouble with teachers or getting into fights. You might notice their being a target of ridicule or 'teasing'. Discriminate between positive and friendly teasing, which is humorous and received in the spirit of a joke, and nasty, malicious teasing that only one person finds funny.

A student's academic performance might drop or they might have an increased number of absentee days. They might withdraw from friendship groups or be more isolated and you might notice differences in where they sit, have lunch or go at break times; for instance, they may ask to stay in a classroom or linger in the library at break or lunchtime.

WHY DO SOME YOUNG PEOPLE BULLY OTHERS?

Research has identified a number of reasons as to why young people bully. Some may bully or engage in other forms of aggressive behaviour for the following reasons:

- So as not to be left out of their peer group.
- To gain social status during childhood and adolescence.
- Because they are influenced by their families and have witnessed or experienced this type of behaviour themselves.
- Making themselves feel better.
- As a way to get what they want.
- To try to impose conformity on another student.
- Because it seems like fun.

Many students are not aware or have not thought much about the harm they are doing. Some are relatively lacking in empathy or compassion.

In the case of cyberbullying, the 'disinhibition effect' operates, i.e. there is a sense that they are anonymous online and this can create the illusion they are not subject to others' judgement, social disapproval or the fear of punishment. Young people who engage in cyberbullying often give as their reasons 'wanting to make themselves feel good' and being able to 'be someone else online'.

Research has shown that most young people who engage in traditional bullying also engage in cyberbullying and vice versa.

SOCIAL NORMS, POWER AND BULLYING

In social groups, people are often expected to look and behave in certain ways in accordance with prevailing social norms. These norms exist within student groups and within schools as a whole. The school's norms can sometimes be influenced – ideally in a positive way – by teachers and other adults.

Student group norms and opinions about which students are of 'greater' social status spring from the values about power and social status observable in wider society. This process happens as children and young people absorb and replicate the norms, values and prejudices of the school and/or the wider community (as the two may not be the same).

Sometimes, students who do not fit in with 'acceptable' social norms are more likely to be bullied. Bullying may also be used to determine the 'in group' and keep those the group identifies as 'different' out. Students can use bullying to enforce or 'police' social norms about appearance or behaviour; for instance, bullying focused on gender roles for boys and girls is common in early high school. Girls or boys whose clothing or behaviour does not fit in with the gender 'norms' of their peer group can be subjected to insults, insinuations or rumours about their sexual preference or activity.

WHAT CAN PARENTS/CARERS DO?

As a guiding principle, always encourage children and young people to act respectfully, kindly, in a friendly way and to accept – value – differences and to try to see things from another person's point of view. If they develop empathy for others when they are young, they are less likely to grow up with unhealthy attitudes of arrogance and superiority.

Children sometimes bully or are involved in bullying situations because of negative peer pressure. Discuss with them ways to resist this sort of pressure and give them words to say like, 'Sorry, but I'm not that kind of person'.

Teach young people to manage conflict and disagreement and model this yourself at home because children and young people watch and imitate your behaviour. Research shows that bullying behaviour starts early – often in the home. Always communicate that bullying behaviour is unacceptable and that it must stop straightaway. If a child tries to justify their actions by blaming the child who is being bullied ('they deserved it'), don't accept this. No child deserves to be bullied.

You've observed some of the signs. You've remembered that the bullying has happened because a relationship went wrong and that it's usually best to repair that relationship in its social setting.

You're having a conversation about this with your child or adolescent.

- Congratulate them on coming to talk to you about bullying. Reassure them it's not their fault.
- Listen. Try to hear the whole story without interrupting. Be empathetic and calm and show you understand what they are saying. They might need to tell their story more than once.
- You could experience very understandable emotions of your own – this story might bring up events from your past. Try not to let these (anger, distress, etc.) show. Your feelings can increase those of the child or make it worse for them. They might even prevent your child from coming to you another time.

- Remind them it's normal to feel hurt, that it's *never* okay to be bullied and that the situation won't just go away.
- Don't suggest they are weak or should be able to stand up to the bullying.
- Find out what you can about the events: note what, when and where the bullying occurred, who was involved, how often and if anybody else witnessed it.
- Don't offer to confront the young person or their parents yourself. Usually, this makes things worse.
- Ask your child what *they* would like to happen. Often all they want is for the bullying to stop. They know if you insist on the perpetrator being punished, it will probably be worse for them in the end.
- Encourage your child not to fight back, but coach them to use neutral or, if appropriate, joking language in response. Help them explore other possible responses, e.g. 'fogging', a technique where the child or young person calmly agrees or acknowledges what the bullying person says without getting angry, defensive or upset.
- Encourage them not to stay and watch or encourage bullying.
- Explain it's safer to avoid people, places or situations that could expose them to further bullying.
- Contact the school to seek help on how to work together to address the situation. It's best not to start by blaming teachers for failing to keep your child safe. Your child may not have told them about the situation. Give them time to investigate. Ensure that they get back to you and make an appointment to check on what has/will happen.
- Think more broadly about your child getting involved in other activities (e.g., drama, dance, sport, or youth groups) so their friendship group is more diverse.
- If the school doesn't help and your child continues to be bullied, explore other avenues, such as informing the educational jurisdiction responsible for the school (Local

Education Authority or relevant religious organisation) or, if you decide that the only option is to take your child away from the school, communicate this to the school and relevant authorities.

- If there are ongoing psychological problems, you might consider seeking professional help. Check with the British Psychological Society's Directory of Chartered Psychologists for reputable practitioners in your area.

WHAT IF A CHILD IS BULLYING OTHER CHILDREN?

- Stay calm. Focus on the behaviour, rather than the child.
- Make sure your child knows bullying behaviour is inappropriate and why.
- Try to understand the reasons why your child has behaved in this way and look for ways to address problems. It may be because they are being bullied in another situation.
- Encourage your child to look at it from the other's perspective – for example, 'How would you feel if …'
- Help your child think of alternative paths of action.
- Provide appropriate boundaries for their behaviour.
- Work with the school to solve the problem. (Many schools now use restorative approaches. The students involved in the bullying situation have a chance to look at the issues. The student who has been bullying has to confront the person they have bullied and look for ways to repair the damage they have caused to the other person and restore their relationship.)
- Children need to find ways of managing their relationships more positively than through dominance, control or exclusion. Teaching conflict resolution and social/emotional skills can be helpful.
- Look candidly at behaviour within your family. Children copy their role models.

WHAT USEFUL ADVICE CAN WE GIVE TO YOUNG PEOPLE WHO ARE BEING BULLIED?

It is important that those who interact with young people are alert to the changes mentioned above and prepared to initiate a conversation about what is troubling them. As we discussed above, they often will not tell an adult what's going on if they are being bullied. They can feel as though this is 'dobbing', or that the adult will either not change the situation or will make it worse. It is very easy to make things worse by insisting that punishment is used: often all a bullied person wants is for the behaviour to stop.

Here are some things you can tell children and young people:

- Keep a record of what happened.
- Tell someone – even if the young person doesn't think it will help. If no one knows, they can't do anything! Just talking about a situation can help put it into perspective. Tell them to talk to a friend, a trusted teacher or a parent/carer who will take the situation seriously.
- Don't ignore it. It will not go away.
- Act unimpressed, pretend not to notice if they're excluded, or if the bullying is verbal, say something like 'Yeah, whatever', or 'Oh, okay'.
- Pretend to agree with them: 'Yep, that's what I'm like, all right', or 'Yeah, my hair is definitely red. Tried dyeing it, but green just didn't suit me'.
- Walk away.
- If they want anonymous advice, Childline (0800 1111) is free and they do not have to give their name.
- Look for other friendships in or out of school.
- Get involved in school clubs or activities where they will be safe.
- If the abuse is physical, the police might have to be called. If they retaliate physically, they could find themselves in trouble for bullying.

Some bullying can be very covert and subtle and not easily identified by teachers. Let the school know if you become aware of possible bullying situations that involve children in other families.

Bullying is a relationship problem, requiring relationship solutions including targeting aggressive behaviour, social skills and problem-solving skills. Ensuring respectful, open and trusting relationships are modelled in the home is the first and most important step in addressing bullying behaviour.

WHAT CAN SCHOOLS DO?

Schools now understand that freedom from bullying and other forms of aggression and harassment is a basic human right and they take their role in its prevention and management very seriously. Schools in many countries are required to have policies that address the issue. Bullying of all kinds can affect students' wellbeing and academic success. When schools fail to address bullying and other negative behaviours systematically, quickly and consistently, teachers' work environments can also become toxic or 'abusive'. Headteachers and teachers who model bullying behaviours can expect to see these replicated in their students. Schools that do not effectively prevent and manage bullying can become places where the more powerful dominate the less powerful.

Schools therefore have a critical role in creating a positive school climate that fosters equality and inclusion. Schools can help to prevent bullying by directly addressing the concepts of power, equality and inequality with students through curriculum, and by supporting student involvement in and connectedness to the school.

Despite the efforts of schools to enhance wellbeing, prevent and effectively address bullying, we know that outcomes vary considerably, even between schools with similar populations. School-based factors are therefore important. Research points to the effectiveness of both proactive and reactive actions. Experts advocate both social educational initiatives and improved ways of intervening in cases to bring about constructive changes in the behaviour of this small, but very important, group.

Schools are pivotal in affecting individual behaviour and influencing broader social change. Whole-school strategies to break up rigid social hierarchies can help to reduce power struggles and the competition for social status. Within a school climate that promotes inclusion and respectful behaviour as the 'norm', bullying is much less likely to happen. These efforts are supported most effectively by robust and collaboratively developed policies endorsed and supported by leadership.

This comprises:

- A **universal whole-school approach**, which involves taking a long-term, multi-faceted approach rather than focusing on one single component.
- A whole-school proactive policy addressing student wellbeing and all forms of bullying in terms of: procedures; training; reporting; thorough investigation; monitoring through surveys; employing evidence-informed and evaluated implementations.
- A positive school environment providing safety, security and support for students and promoting positive relationships and wellbeing.
- A focus on promoting pro-social skills and competencies throughout the age groups.
- Teacher understandings and competencies:
  - Clear recognition of what does and does not comprise a bullying situation.
  - Knowledge of how to respond and responsibility to do so.
  - Effective classroom management and classroom rules to ensure that classrooms are safe spaces for young people.
  - Effective non-hostile and non-punitive behaviour-management methods consistently applied.
- An increased awareness of bullying in the school community through curriculum, assemblies, focus days and student-owned plans and activities.
- Involvement of young people in building the safe, secure climate that enhances wellbeing.
- School–family–community partnerships.

Dr Ken Rigby, who is a leading expert and researcher on bullying, endorses proactive approaches while also recognising that schools sometimes have to use reactive strategies in dealing with bullying.

These can include:

- direct sanctions (for example, suspension, exclusion). In very serious cases, the police may have to be involved
- school tribunals
- serious talks
- bullying prevention in Positive Behaviour Support (PBIS)
- strengthening the victim
- mediation
- restorative approaches
- the Support Group Method
- the Method of Shared Concern.

Selection of the appropriate response will depend on the severity of the incident, whether it was a group or individual offence, if the perpetrator was remorseful, the training of the teacher responding and the age of the student.

> Teachers and others who work with young people need to receive professional learning about bullying: what it is, how to recognise it, how to respond at the time of the incident and how to manage it over time.

More information and advice is contained on Dr Ken Rigby's website: www.kenrigby.net

WHAT CAN TEACHERS DO?

A teacher's role is pivotal not only in responding to bullying but also in effectively preventing it. Students respond better to teachers they like, trust and respect.

Teachers can take some relatively simple actions to prevent and effectively address bullying by:

- Developing positive and respectful relationships: learn one or two details about your students' lives to ensure you have something to talk to them about. It will give them the sense that you value them.
- Being there is one of the most important things teachers can do. Leaving the classroom creates ideal conditions for bullying to prosper. I've seen teachers go to collect photocopies and all hell break loose after they've left.
- Creating positive expectations for their behaviour and achievement.
- Establishing a 'no putdowns' rule.
- Greeting students at the door of your classroom at the beginning of the day/lesson.
- Contacting families with good news about students' progress or behaviour.

To respond effectively to bullying, you should:

- Never ignore a bullying situation. Address bullying wherever you see it, in line with the school's explicit policies and guidelines. It will be easier and more effective to do so as you already have a relationship with students.
- Stay calm.
- Have a quiet talk to bullying young people; explain that their behaviour isn't acceptable and if there is no change, action will be taken in line with school policy.
- Call out bullying behaviour – make it clear that you know what is going on, what the behaviour is intended to do – i.e. put another student down or impress others – and be clear that you will not allow it to continue.
- Allow students to keep their dignity even when they have been involved in bullying or you have to discipline them.

Correct them in a private location. Avoid communicating negative judgements, low expectations or disgust. Treat each student fairly and equitably and ensure they know this.

WHAT DOES A SAFE, BULLY-FREE SCHOOL LOOK LIKE?

The message that bullying behaviour is unacceptable is communicated consistently and firmly. Policies clearly outlining rights, responsibilities and procedures for reporting concerns about bullying are strongly communicated in jargon-free language and people know about them. Students have many opportunities to build on their strengths and receive recognition. Classrooms are orderly, but buzz with interest and activity. Students are often working in groups and their work is on display. Friendliness and respect, lack of suspicion and a willingness to help are demonstrated by all. Teachers and students speak to each other in a friendly and respectful way. The school works hard to connect people to each other and to the school, and social relationships and interactions are characterised by caring, acceptance of differences and respect for others and the school. Conflict management processes are in place and focus on restoring relationships rather than punishment. If bullying situations arise, teachers are skilled in the use of management strategies, which they immediately and effectively employ. Suspension rates are low. There is minimal rubbish or graffiti. At break times, students have plenty of options for both active and passive activities and engage in these cooperatively. The students know they're safe there.

> Bullying is everyone's responsibility and needs collaboration from parents, schools, health workers and communities to prevent and manage it.

Acknowledgments

Many thanks to NCAB members Ken Rigby, Marilyn Campbell and Helen McGrath for their support with the writing of this chapter.

Author biography

Sandra Craig is Manager of the National Centre Against Bullying (NCAB) at The Alannah & Madeline Foundation. After a career in secondary schools, she taught briefly at Deakin University and went on to be involved in research into bullying policy and practice. She has written submissions to government and various publications, and been involved in educational programme development.

www.ncab.org.au

See also:

Chapter 4: Anxiety in Young People
Chapter 5: Depression in Young People

Recommended websites:

National Bullying Helpline: www.nationalbullyinghelpline.co.uk
Childline: www.childline.org.uk
NHS: www.nhs.uk/livewell/bullying
Bullying UK: www.bullying.co.uk
BulliesOut: bulliesout.com
Anti-Bullying Alliance: www.anti-bullyingalliance.og.uk
Kidscape: www.kidscape.org.uk
Ken Rigby: www.kenrigby.net

Further reading:

Alsaker, FV 2001, *Peer Harassment in School. The Plight of the Vulnerable and Victimized* (JG Juvoven, Ed.), The Guildford Press, New York.

Barker, EB 2008, 'Predictive Validity and Early Predictors of Peer-Victimization Trajectories in Preschool', *Arch Gen Psychiatry*, vol. 65 no. 10, pp 1185–1192.

Casas, JW 2006, 'Early parenting and children's relational and physical aggression in the preschool and home contexts', Psychology Faculty Publications.

Cross, D, Shaw, T, Hearn, L, Epstein, M, Monks, H, Lester, L, & Thomas, L 2009, *Australian covert cullying prevalence study (ACBPS)* Child Health Promotion Research Centre, Edith Cowan University, Perth.

Durlak, JA, Weissberg, RP, Dymnicki, AB, Taylor, RD & Schellinger, KB 2011, 'The Impact of Enhancing Students' Social and Emotional Learning: A Meta-Analysis of School-based Universal Interventions', *Child Development*, vol. 82, pp 405–432.

Espelage, D, & De La Rue, L 2011, 'School bullying: its nature and ecology', *International Journal of Adolescent Medicine and Health*, vol. 24, no. 1, pp 3–10.

Espelage, D, Basile, KC, De La Rue, L, & Hamburger, ME 2015, 'Longitudinal Associations Among Bullying, Homophobic Teasing, and Sexual Violence Perpetration Among Middle School Students', *Journal of Interpersonal Violence,* vol. 30, pp 2541–2561.

Hinduja, SC & Patchin, JW 2012, 'Cyberbullying: Neither an epidemic nor a rarity', *European Journal of Developmental Psychology*, vol. 9, no. 5.

McGrath, H & Noble, T (Eds) 2006, *Bullying Solutions – evidence-based approaches to bullying in Australian schools*, Pearson Longman, Australia.

McGrath, H & Noble, T 2003, *BounceBack! Teacher's Resource Book*, Pearson Longman, Australia.

McGrath, H (ed), *The Important Role of Parents in the Development and Maintenance of a Safe & Supportive School Community* – Handout Notes.

Nation, M, Vieno, A, Perkins, DD & Santinello, M 2008, 'Bullying in schools and a sense of empowerment: An analysis of relationships with parents, friends and teachers', *Journal of Community and Applied Social Psychology*, vol. 18, pp 211–232.

Perren, SA 2006, 'Social behavior and peer relationships of victims, bully-victims, and bullies in kindergarten', *Journal of Child Psychology and Psychiatry*, vol. 47, no. 1, pp 45–57.

Polanin, JR, Espelage, DL & Pigott, TD 2012, 'A meta-analysis of school-based bullying prevention programs' effects on bystander intervention behaviour', *School Psychology Review*, vol. 41, no. 1, p 47.

Rigby, K 2013, 'Bullying in schools and its relation to parenting and family life', *Family Matters*, no. 92, pp 61–67.

Rigby, K 2012, 'Bullying in Schools: Addressing Desires, Not Only Behaviours', *Educational Psychology Review*, vol. 24, pp 339–348.

Rigby, K 2011, 'What can schools do about cases of bullying?' *Pastoral Care in Education*, vol. 29, no. 4, pp 273–285.

Rigby, K 2010, *Bullying Interventions: in schools: six basic approaches*, ACER, Camberwell.

Rigby, K 2002, *New perspectives on bullying*, Jessica Kingsley, London.

Rigby, K & Johnson, K 2016, *The Prevalence and Effectiveness of Anti-Bullying Strategies employed in Australian Schools*, University of South Australia, Adelaide.

Rigby, K, & Smith, PK 2011, 'Is school bullying really on the rise?' *Social Psychology of Education*, vol. 14, no. 4, pp 441–455.

Sanders, D, Pattison, P & Bible, J 2012, 'Legislating "Nice": analysis and assessment of proposed workplace bullying prohibitions', *Southern Law Journal*, vol. XXII.

Smith, PK 2014, *Understanding School Bullying: its nature and prevention strategies*, Sage, London.

Smith, PK, & Ananiadou, K 2003, 'The Nature of School Bullying and the Effectiveness of School-Based Interventions', *Journal of Applied Psychoanalytic Studies*, vol. 5, no. 2.

Ttofi, MM & Farrington, DP 2011, 'Effectiveness of school-based programs to reduce bullying: A systematic and meta-analytic review', *Journal of Experimental Criminology*, vol. 7, pp 27–56.

Vlachou, MA 2011, 'Bully/Victim Problems Among Preschool Children: a Review of Current Research Evidence', *Education Psychology Review*, vol. 23, pp 329–358.

Wilton, C & Campbell, MA 2011, 'An exploration of the reasons why adolescents engage in traditional and cyber bullying', *Journal of Educational Sciences & Psychology*, vol. 1, no. 2, pp 101–109.

Wang, C, Berry, B & Swearer, Susan M 2013, 'The Critical Role of School Climate in Effective Bullying Prevention', *Theory Into Practice*, vol. 52, no. 4.

For more online resources visit:
generationnext.com.au/handbook

4. ANXIETY IN YOUNG PEOPLE

Professor Jennie Hudson & Dr Anna McKinnon

This chapter will provide an overview of anxiety problems in adolescence and is for parents, teachers and other adults who have contact with adolescents who could be experiencing an anxiety disorder. Readers will gain an understanding of what anxiety is, what causes anxiety problems, how to recognise when anxiety becomes a problem, and what to do to receive support.

INTRODUCTION

Anxiety and fear are normal emotions experienced by all young people to differing degrees when faced with a perceived threat or danger. Accompanying these emotions are changes in the body, mind and behaviour that allow a young person to react to danger very quickly. The 'flight or fight response' is the term used to describe the series of changes that happen in the human body automatically when threat/ danger is detected. The brain sends signals to the young person's adrenal glands to release the hormones adrenaline and noradrenaline, which activate the sympathetic nervous system, and send signals to various parts of the body to prepare to 'flight' (i.e. to run away). In children without anxiety this system tends to be activated when faced with real danger. For a child with anxiety, the flight or fight system can be activated when there is no real danger/threat or the chance of danger is exaggerated. This explains why anxiety often occurs in everyday situations and is typically accompanied by a range of physical symptoms like nausea, racing heart, breathlessness, shaking and blushing. It also explains why the most common way a young person reacts when he or she experiences fear or anxiety is to avoid whatever is scaring him or her. By keeping away from the perceived danger, the young person is kept safe in the short term, but in the long term this 'flight' response leads to persistent anxiety as the young person never gets the chance to learn accurate information about avoided situations.

Anxiety symptoms are thought to constitute a disorder when they are experienced more intensely and more often than others, and the symptoms stop a young person from being able to do things others enjoy and getting the most out of life. One in four Australians will, during their lifetime, experience an anxiety disorder. Anxiety disorders are the most common mental health problem diagnosed during adolescence, with at least one in ten young people experiencing anxiety that affects their daily life. The first onset of an anxiety disorder often occurs in early childhood and parents may report that the young person has 'always' been worried or shy. However, in some instances a person who has been emotionally healthy during childhood can develop a debilitating anxiety disorder abruptly during adolescence. Regardless of when the problem started, anxiety disorders have a significant impact on a young person's health and wellbeing. Anxiety disorders can often lead to other mental health problems like depression, suicide or substance abuse. For example, the young person may start to use alcohol or other substances excessively to reduce their anxiety, further complicating the problem.

For many years, anxiety disorders have been under-recognised and often overshadowed by other mental health problems such as attention deficit hyperactivity disorder, eating disorders and even depression. In fact, less than 20 per cent of young people with an anxiety disorder seek treatment. One of the common myths about anxiety is that the young person will grow out of it. While this may be true for some young people, for most, unless they receive treatment, anxiety will continue to interfere with their daily activities and result in subsequent problems throughout their lives.

Without treatment, a young person with an anxiety disorder can experience lifelong suffering, resulting in more sick days, less productivity at work, and less life satisfaction and happiness. Importantly, anxiety disorders respond very well to psychological interventions, and treatments like Cognitive Behavioural Therapy (CBT). The delivery of these interventions during adolescence can significantly improve the young person's wellbeing, academic achievements, and social and family relationships. These findings highlight the importance of intervening to treat anxiety as early as possible, so as to prevent the negative outcomes that could potentially happen in adulthood.

COMMON PRESENTATIONS OF ANXIETY

There are several different types of anxiety disorders that affect young people, including social anxiety, panic, general worry, specific fears (e.g. heights, dogs, transport) or separation fears. A young person may only have one type of anxiety disorder or they may have several different types. The presence of a state of fear, worry or dread that greatly impairs the young person's ability to function normally is common to all anxiety disorders. Furthermore, these fears are accompanied by strong and persistent physiological responses, including difficulty concentrating, stomach aches, headaches, difficulty sleeping and muscle aches. The unique characteristics of these disorders are described as follows.

Social Anxiety: Social anxiety disorder refers to excessive fear and worry in situations where the young person has to interact with other people or be the focus of attention. The socially anxious young person is overly concerned that others will think badly of him/her and that he/she will do something embarrassing. Although social anxiety and an increased focus on 'what others think' is a normal experience during adolescence, a young person with social anxiety may have difficulty making friends, participating in class or social activities, sitting exams, answering questions or talking to others. A young person with social anxiety may experience physical symptoms such as stomach aches, nausea, blushing, or trembling. He/she may appear shy or withdrawn, often speaking quietly or not saying much. Other signs include having difficulty joining in with others, having a limited number of friends and avoiding a range of social situations (e.g. talking on the phone, asking/answering questions in class).

Generalised Anxiety: A young person with generalised anxiety disorder worries about multiple things like their health, schoolwork, getting into trouble at school, performing at school or in sports, family relationships, friendships, money, safety and world events. This worry is experienced as uncontrollable and can't be switched off easily. It is accompanied by a range of physical symptoms like stomach and muscle aches, headaches, feeling irritable, having trouble concentrating and difficulties sleeping. A young person with generalised anxiety may be perfectionistic in their approach to schoolwork and become particularly stressed around exam time. One of the key signs a young person is suffering from generalised anxiety is that he/she asks a lot of repetitive reassurance-seeking questions (e.g. 'What is going to happen?', 'What if...?'). Some young people will often ask lots of questions over and over in a new situation. Generalised anxiety can be missed or overlooked because the young person can be very conscientious at school and the excessive worry is often not observable to others.

Separation Anxiety: Separation anxiety disorder occurs when a young person is excessively fearful about leaving his/her parents or caregivers and worries that something will happen to either the parents or to him/her on separation. Separation anxiety disorder is far less common in adolescence than it is in childhood, but it can still be a problem for some young people. A young person with separation anxiety may not like being left alone and often wants to be with a parent. This means he/she will often avoid school, sleep in the same bed as a parent, and avoid sleepovers or school camps. Other symptoms include stomach aches, excessive worry before separation, and needing to have a parent present when going to sleep.

Panic Disorder and Agoraphobia: Panic attacks can occur in a range of situations (e.g. social situations, exams, being confronted with a scary situation) and involve a sudden rush of fear accompanied by physical feelings such as a racing heart, breathlessness, tightness in the throat or chest, sweating, light-headedness and/or tingling. During a panic attack, a young person may believe that he/she is dying or that something terrible is happening. This is typically a terrifying experience. Panic disorder occurs when these panic attacks seem to come out of the blue and are not connected to another fear like panicking during an exam for fear of failing, or panicking before a performance because of a fear of making a mistake. A young person with panic disorder is very fearful and worries a great deal about having future panic attacks. The fear is of the panic attack specifically ('I am having a heart attack') rather than of the situation (e.g. an exam). Typically, the young person starts avoiding situations in which it might be difficult to escape if a panic attack were to occur (e.g. public transport, school assemblies).

RED FLAGS – WHAT TO LOOK OUT FOR

- Skipping school
- Refusing activities and reluctance to try new activities
- Asking lots of repetitive questions
- Avoiding eye contact
- Blushing, shaking or mumbling answers in social situations
- Becoming sick right before an event or test or performance
- Slow to complete activities
- Being on high alert for danger
- Always thinking the worst
- Distress following changes in routine
- Avoiding certain people, places or situations
- Not wanting to be left alone

WHAT CAUSES ANXIETY?

There are biological, environmental and individual factors that place a young person at risk of developing an anxiety disorder. There is a moderate degree of heritability of anxiety disorders. About 30 to 40 per cent of the variance in anxiety symptoms is genetically determined. If a young person is anxious, it's likely that others in the child's family also have experienced anxiety and/or depression. A young person may not inherit the same type of anxiety as the parent or grandparent. There are also environmental reasons that may cause anxiety disorders to develop. Young people learn a great deal about what to be fearful of from their parents or others in their social world, either through watching what others are fearful of or by hearing from their parents or friends (e.g. 'stay away from spiders', 'don't go near the edge', 'everyone is going to laugh'). Some young people are also more temperamentally vulnerable, that is, they may be born with a tendency to avoid new situations or are temperamentally shy.

One of the main reasons anxiety disorders persist is because the natural response to a potentially scary situation is to stay away from it. The problem is that the young person's solution to the problem – to avoid – actually maintains the disorder. Avoiding the situation means the young person misses out on opportunities to learn accurate information about the situation, such as 'nothing bad happened' or 'I can cope'. Avoidance of the situation can include skipping school or refusing party invitations. Sometimes avoidance can be quite subtle, such as needing to always hold a special object when sitting an exam or attending a party but not talking very much to people or leaving early. The outcome is the same: the young person never learns that the situation is safe and that they can handle the situation without these supports. Once avoidance has become persistent, fears can become quite chronic, and pushing them to confront fears must be handled in a graded fashion (i.e. develop a step-by-step plan).

Sometimes parents or people in the young person's life can unintentionally exacerbate the anxiety by accommodating the anxiety. For example, parents allow the child to skip important activities, or parents complete certain activities that the young person struggles with or may refuse to do. Sometimes parents may also try to reduce the young person's stress by helping them too much or rushing in to quickly come to their aid. These behaviours help to maintain the young person's anxiety and prevent them from learning critical information about the safety of the situation and the young person's true ability to cope with the situation.

DOS AND DON'TS FOR PARENTS AND CARERS

Don't

- Dismiss or ignore the young person's fear.
- Push the child to face situations they don't want to face.
- Constantly reassure the young person.
- Do everything for them (e.g. asking a question on behalf of the child when they will not ask it).
- Rush to the young person's assistance in vulnerable situations before they exhibit signs of anxiety.
- Criticise the child.
- Label the child as 'shy' or 'anxious'.

Do

- Listen and acknowledge the young person's fear.
- Use the words the young person uses to describe his/her anxiety.
- Encourage the young person to collect evidence for his/her worried thoughts and ask questions rather than reassure. For example, rather than saying, 'Nothing bad will happen' ask, 'What happened last time?'
- Gently encourage the young person to face his/her fear in a gradual fashion as this is the key to overcoming anxiety.
- Use incentives and positive reinforcement to motivate the young person to face their fears.

HOW TO COMMUNICATE EFFECTIVELY ABOUT ANXIETY

Although stigma around mental illness has improved over the last decade, young people can still feel guilty or ashamed about their worries and fears, and hence experience difficulties talking about them. Some people see having a mental health problem as a weakness and this can make it difficult to acknowledge the problem, particularly for adolescent males. It is critical that adults provide a safe and non-judgemental space for a young person to talk about his/her experiences. A young person needs to know he/she will be understood and listened to without judgement. A young person may not identify with the words *anxiety*, *feeling scared* or *fearful*, but may report feeling 'stressed' as this, for some, may be a more socially acceptable term. Other young people may have a wide and expressive vocabulary for their fears. This can be very person specific. Importantly, when communicating about anxiety it's best to use language and words consistent with a young person's vocabulary. For example, if a young person talks about 'feeling stressed' rather than anxious or worried, then use the word 'stress' instead.

WHAT IS THE DIFFERENCE BETWEEN NORMAL ANXIETY AND A DISORDER?

It can be difficult to know the difference between anxiety that would be considered normal and anxiety that requires treatment. One way to think about this is on a continuum with low levels of anxiety on one end and extreme anxiety at the other end. For most people anxiety on a daily basis is low and may peak at different stressful periods (such as exams, just before a school presentation or school trip). But if anxiety is occurring daily or more days than not, or it is stopping the young person from participating in activities their peers are involved in, or causing the family or the young person a great deal of distress, then we would consider it problematic.

WHEN TO SEEK HELP

In deciding whether a young person needs help, please consider the following questions:

- Is the young person's anxiety stopping him/her from doing things they want to be able to do or interfering with friendships, schoolwork or family life?
- Is the anxiety occurring more often and more intensely compared with peers?

If the answer to one of these questions is 'yes', then consider seeking help.

Professional help

There are several options for seeking professional help, including: a specialist anxiety clinic or online services (see Recommended websites at the end of the chapter), a school counsellor, GP or paediatrician, psychiatrist or the local community mental health team. Currently, the best evidence for the first line of treatment of anxiety disorders is Cognitive Behavioural Therapy (CBT). CBT provides skills to help the young person collect evidence for their anxious thoughts and increases their ability to cope independently. CBT includes gradual exposure, which involves gently encouraging the young person to face the feared situations. Evidence-based guidelines recommend CBT, and this can be delivered in a variety of formats, from individual, family (e.g. with parents) or group therapy. There is strong evidence to support face-to-face delivery with a qualified therapist and emerging evidence to support the efficacy of therapist-guided online CBT (particularly as an initial step). Although not recommended as a first line of treatment, antidepressant medications are sometimes used when symptoms are severe or CBT has not been successful. There is also some initial evidence that combining CBT and medication leads to enhanced outcomes, particularly in severe cases. There is currently not sufficient evidence to support the use of mindfulness therapies for young people experiencing anxiety.

TAKE-HOME MESSAGES FOR PARENTS

- Early intervention is important.
- Encourage the young person's bravery.
- Encourage the young person to face their fears in a gradual fashion.
- Encourage and support the young person's independence and allow them to make their own choices. Rather than rushing in to help the young person or finishing his/her assignment, stand back and ask, 'What can my child learn from doing this on his/her own?'
- Provide a safe and non-judgemental space for the young person to talk about their fears and worries.

TAKE-HOME MESSAGES FOR TEACHERS AND SCHOOL COUNSELLORS/YOUTH WORKERS

- CBT has strong evidence in support of its efficacy.
- Gradual exposure is a key component to successful treatment. If you are not conducting exposures (facing fears), preferably in a gradual way, the treatment is unlikely to be effective.
- Use incentives and positive reinforcement to motivate the young person to face their fears.

Authors' biographies

Professor Jennie Hudson is the Director, Centre for Emotional Health, Macquarie University. Jennie's research focuses on understanding the factors that contribute to children's emotional health and improving interventions available to children experiencing anxiety disorders. Jennie is a co-author of the Cool Kids programme and the books *Treating anxious children: An evidence-based approach* and *Psychopathology and the Family*.

Dr Anna McKinnon is a clinical psychologist at the Centre for Emotional Health Clinic. Her research investigates the cognitive, behavioural, emotional and biological factors maintaining psychological disorders in the aftermath of trauma.

See also:
Chapter 5: Depression in Young People
Chapter 18: What is Resilience and How to Do It
Chapter 20: Using Positive Psychology
Chapter 21: Food, Mood and Mental Health

Recommended websites:
Mind: www.mind.org.uk
NHS: www.nhs.uk/conditions/generalised-anxiety-disorder.uk.org
Anxiety UK: www.anxietyuk.org.uk
Mental Health Foundation: www.mentalhealth.org.uk
NHS: www.nhs.uk/Livewell/youth-mental-health
The Mix: www.themix.org.uk/mental-health/anxiety-ocd-and-phobias

Further reading:
Rapee, RM, Schniering, CA & Hudson, JL 2009, 'Anxiety disorders during childhood and adolescence: Origins and treatment', Annual Review of Clinical Psychology, vol. 5, pp 335–365.
Rapee, RM, Wignall, A, Hudson, JL & Schniering, CA 2000, Treating anxiety in children: An evidence-based approach, New Harbinger Publications, Oakland.

 For more online resources visit:
generationnext.com.au/handbook

5. DEPRESSION IN YOUNG PEOPLE

Dr Bridianne O'Dea & Dr Aliza Werner-Seidler

This chapter will provide an overview of depression in adolescence. Readers will gain an understanding of what depression is, how to recognise it and what to do for support.

INTRODUCTION

At any given time, approximately 6 per cent of Australian adults have depression. By the age of eighteen years, up to 20 per cent of teenagers will have experienced a depressive episode.

Worldwide, depression is a major public health issue. It is a mental illness characterised by overwhelming sadness, a low mood and lack of hope for the future. It is very common in adults (one in five women, and one in eight men), and carries the greatest burden of disease. There are certain times in life when people are more at risk of developing depression. Adolescence is one of these times. Up to half of all mental health issues, including depression, show first signs between the ages of twelve and eighteen years. The risk of depression rises substantially throughout adolescence. This is because adolescence is a time of great change in both the mind and body, and also the social world. During the teenage years, young people become more independent and place a huge importance on their friendships and social connections. Brain maturation, including puberty and changes in thinking processes, result in changes to the brain circuits that expose the brain to higher levels of stress. Combined, these factors lead to higher risk of depression. Among early adolescents, the rate of depression is approximately 5 per cent, but by the age of eighteen years, up to 20 per cent of young people will have experienced a depressive episode. An earlier onset of depression is likely to result in a more severe experience of depression, including more depressive episodes throughout life.

Depression affects more than just a teenager's mood. It can lead to serious social and educational impairments, including social withdrawal, reduced academic achievement, and trouble with concentration and memory. Adolescents with depression are more likely to reduce their school attendance, often being absent for twenty days more than their healthy peers. Depression is also associated with an increased rate of substance use including tobacco and other drugs, as well as obesity and other risky behaviour. Depression is also a major risk factor for suicide.

Depression often co-occurs alongside other mental health issues and physical health issues. Two-thirds of adolescents with depression have at least one other mental health issue, and up to 15 per cent have two or more. Adolescents with depression are six to twelve times more likely to have anxiety, four to eleven times more likely to have a disruptive behaviour disorder, and three to six times more likely to have a substance misuse problem than their peers who are not depressed. Depression can also complicate eating disorders, autism spectrum disorders, attention deficit hyperactivity disorders as well as other behavioural issues.

The good news is that effective treatments for depression are available, and prevention and early intervention efforts are key. As such, it is important for parents, teachers and other adults to recognise depression early and act quickly to avoid lifelong adversities. This chapter will help you to do just that.

WHAT IS DEPRESSION?

Depression is a mental illness that is generally characterised by the following:

- A depressed mood that is present for most of the day, and almost every day.
- A loss of interest or pleasure in usually enjoyable activities.
- Decreased energy and feelings of fatigue.
- Loss of confidence and self-esteem.
- Unreasonable feelings of guilt and self-loathing.
- Thoughts of death, suicide or self-harm.
- Inability to concentrate or think clearly.
- Problems falling asleep and staying asleep.
- Changes in appetite and weight.

It can be hard for people to tell the difference between 'natural' sadness and depression. This can be particularly hard during adolescence, due to the normal development changes that occur during this time. Unlike natural sadness, depression in adolescence is characterised specifically by:

- A noticeable change in mood that is quite severe, and lasts for two weeks or more.
- No longer finding favourite activities enjoyable.
- Trouble concentrating, staying focused, and getting schoolwork done.
- Disruptions to daily life, like increased friction in relationships with family and friends.
- Avoidance of normal activities like going to school or socialising.
- Spending more time alone and away from people, such as in their bedroom.
- Sleeping much more or much less than usual.
- Feeling more hungry than usual, or not feeling hungry at all.
- No plans for the future, disinterested in future planning.

One of the most important ways to distinguish between natural sadness and depression is the extent to which these thoughts and feelings are interfering with everyday life, or the extent to which they are distressing. For example, if these thoughts and feelings get in the way of a young person completing their schoolwork or getting on with their friends, and last for more than two weeks, it's a sign that it's probably something more than just natural sadness.

Depression can make a young person feel like they are unlikely to get better. For some, this can lead to thoughts that they might be better off dead, or thoughts about hurting themselves. Young people can be very ashamed and guilty about feeling this way and can start to feel very scared. But these thoughts are common and it is a sign that extra support is needed. These thoughts should always be taken seriously.

WHAT CAUSES DEPRESSION?

There is no one cause of depression. This is because there are many individual, family and social risks that are highly related to each other, and mental illness is a complex issue. There are, however, some known factors which may place a young person at greater risk of experiencing depression. These include:

Gender: The risk of depression is higher among adolescent females than males (approximately twice as high). The reasons for this are not fully understood. Some propose that the risk of depression is linked closely to hormonal stress in the body, which places females at greater risk as they enter puberty earlier than their male peers. And although depression is more common among females, males are still affected, and recognising depression in boys is equally important.

Family history: Some young people will have a genetic vulnerability to developing mental illness like depression. Young people with parents who have depression are three to four times more likely to experience depression when compared to their peers without depressed parents. Both genes and non-inherited factors contribute to these risks. To date, there has not been a single gene that is known to increase the susceptibility of depression.

Stressful events: Prolonged stressful events like trouble at home (e.g. parental conflict, divorce), peer conflict (e.g. fights with friends or bullying) or trauma (e.g. abuse) can place an adolescent at risk of depression. Exams are especially stressful periods, particularly final school year exams, which can increase risk.

Substance use: Some types of drugs, including alcohol and cannabis, can have the effect of making people feel down and depressed.

Other causes: Depression can also be caused by or related to other things, such as the effects of medication or a physical health problem or injury. Depression can also happen for no reason at all. A trained professional like a psychologist or doctor can help figure out what might be triggering depression. That is why it is very important to seek help. Struggling alone can prolong the depression. It is important also to remember that you may never identify the cause. This can be confusing for the young person and the family. In the same way that there is often no cause for physical illnesses, the same is true for depression. It is important that you work through this with a trained professional, and it is often a relief for young people to discover that their depression is no fault of their own.

WHAT PROTECTS AGAINST DEPRESSION?

Many young people who are at high risk of depression do not go on to develop the disorder. There are factors that are protective against developing depression. High-quality interpersonal relationships with friends, family and other adults can protect against depression. Young people with higher levels of social support (e.g. feeling that they are loved and cared for by their family and friends) are at a lower risk of developing depression. Relationships characterised by warmth, acceptance, low hostility and low parental control are important for the prevention of depression. Other protective factors include emotion regulation ability, healthy coping mechanisms (like sport, exercise and social interaction) and positive thinking styles.

WHAT ARE THE WARNING SIGNS OF DEPRESSION?

There are a number of signs and symptoms of depression, but everyone experiences this illness differently so it is not always easy to tell. Here are some common red flags that a young person may be going through a tough time:

- Difficulty concentrating, remembering details, making decisions
- A feeling of weariness, tiredness, or lack of energy
- Feelings of excessive or inappropriate guilt
- Having a low sense of worth
- Feeling without hope
- Feelings of pessimism
- Sadness
- Irritability, anger, or hostility
- Frequent crying
- Withdrawal from friends and family
- Loss of interest in activities
- Complete loss of motivation
- Poor school performance
- Changes in eating, such as overeating or restrictive eating
- Changes in sleep habits, such as staying awake at night and sleeping during the day
- Apathy towards life
- Complaints of physical pains, like headaches or stomach aches that have no medical cause
- Irresponsible behaviour – forgetting obligations, being late for classes, skipping school or rebellious behaviour.

Depression carries a high risk of suicide. Young people with depression often experience thoughts that they would be better off dead, or thoughts about harming or killing themselves. This is part of the disorder, and requires serious and special attention. Experiencing depression in adolescence can compound what is an already difficult time. Depression can often make problems seem overwhelming and unbearable. This is often when young people are most at risk of suicide.

THE WARNING SIGNS OF SUICIDE

- Expressing hopelessness for the future.
- Giving up on one's self, talking as if no one cares.
- Preparing for death by writing goodbye letters.
- Starting to use drugs or alcohol or other sleeping medications to relieve mental anguish.
- Thoughts of dying, as well as making a plan, and attempting suicide.
- Self-harming behaviour, such as cutting.

If these behaviours or thoughts emerge, it is important to seek help immediately. Anybody who expresses suicidal thoughts or intentions should be taken very seriously. Do not hesitate to call your local suicide hotline, such as Samaritans or Childline, immediately. You can also contact your local hospital or emergency services line if there is imminent risk. In addition, seek help from your general practitioner or mental health professional when this occurs.

HOW IS DEPRESSION DIAGNOSED?

If you think someone you know may be depressed, then seeking help from a trained professional will assist in confirming a diagnosis, or provide an alternative explanation for what is going on. This is done in order to work out what treatment is most appropriate. When seeking professional help, the clinician will typically undertake a diagnostic assessment. This consists of sensitive, empathetic questioning about how the young person has been feeling lately, the duration and severity of these feelings, and whether there has been any interruption to their daily activities like school and work. The clinician will also ask about feelings of suicide and death. There are two main classification systems that are used by health professionals to diagnose and treat depression.

These systems use similar diagnostic criteria and work somewhat like a checklist. The clinical and diagnostic features of depression are broadly similar in adolescents and adults. The core symptoms of depression include:

- Depressed, irritable, or cranky mood present for most of the day, and almost every day.
- Loss of interest or pleasure in activities most of the day, nearly every day.

Other associated symptoms include:

- Loss of confidence or self-esteem.
- Unreasonable feelings of self-reproach or excessive and inappropriate guilt.
- Recurrent thoughts of death or suicide, or any suicidal behaviour (including self-harm).
- Diminished ability to think or concentrate.
- Changes in movement, coordination and reflexes.
- Agitation.
- Sleep disturbance.
- Change in appetite with corresponding change in weight (can be loss or gain).

To receive a diagnosis of depression, at least one of the two cardinal symptoms (depressed or irritable mood, loss of interest or pleasure) is required, and a total of four other symptoms need to be reported.

Once this assessment is complete, the clinician will discuss the results with the young person and, when appropriate, with their parents or guardians. Depression can be mild, moderate or severe, depending on the constellation and number of symptoms, as well as the degree to which they impact on daily life. The health professional will also assess other factors, such as physical illnesses or injuries, to rule out any possible other illness. They will also ask about any recent deaths because bereavement due to loss is different to depression. Once a diagnosis is confirmed, the clinician will then move to discuss appropriate treatments. If a clinician is unable to determine a diagnosis, it is likely they will refer the young person to a more suitable health professional such as a psychologist or psychiatrist.

It is important to note that depression is often not picked up among adolescents, due to the higher level of irritability, which is sometimes labelled by parents and friends as 'adolescent moodiness'. The fluctuating pattern of symptoms, which is sometimes due to hormones, is often referred to as the 'emotional roller-coaster', which also makes it difficult for parents and other adults to recognise a mental health issue. Depression may also be missed due to a tendency to focus only on the primary presenting problem. For example, a young person who refuses to attend school or has a decline in academic performance, other behavioural problems or substance use, may not be flagged as someone experiencing depression when this may be the case.

MYTHS ABOUT DEPRESSION

Here are some common myths about depression in youth:

- Only people who are weak or not resilient enough get depression.
- Depression isn't a real illness – it's just a bad attitude.
- Depression will go away on its own with time.
- One can 'snap out' of depression.
- Antidepressants are addictive and bad for you.

All of these myths are simply not true. It is important that you reassure young people, their parents and carers that depression is a serious mental illness that requires proper treatment. If you have questions or concerns, it is always best to seek help from a trained mental health professional.

WHAT TO DO IF YOU THINK SOMEONE IS DEPRESSED

If you think someone you know may be depressed, the most important thing you can offer them is your care and support. Here are a few simple suggestions on what to do when someone you know may be depressed:

- Create a safe and supportive place where you can chat to them about how they are feeling. Be a supportive listener by not forcing them, being patient and compassionate. Ensure you give them the time that is needed.
- Encourage the person to seek professional help. You can suggest taking them to their doctor, calling a telephone line with them, or arranging a meeting for them with a mental health professional. If the person seems reluctant to seek help, be supportive.
- Keep checking with the person to see how they are feeling.
- Ask them if they have been feeling like hurting themselves or having thoughts of suicide. If yes, encourage them to seek professional help. If the person isn't ready, suggest they call a helpline, which can put into place a safety plan. If it's an emergency, don't hesitate to call 999 or 112.
- Try to schedule some time to do enjoyable activities together, like socialising, going out, films or games.
- Look after yourself – know your limits. Take care of yourself so that you can stay strong and positive. Don't go beyond your expertise, instead refer on.

Always remember that depression is an illness that needs treatment from professionals. Therefore, while talking to family and friends will help, depression is a serious issue that needs to be addressed by professionals who have experience working with depression. Given that depression is linked to poor outcomes across the lifespan, it is important to get professional help early, even if a parent or carer feels that the issue is only mild.

HOW IS DEPRESSION TREATED?

Most importantly, there are effective treatments for depression in adolescents. One such treatment is Cognitive Behavioural Therapy (CBT), which is a psychological therapy aimed at targeting the links between negative thinking, emotion and behaviour. It is most effective when delivered by a trained professional, which is usually a clinical psychologist or a registered psychologist with specialist CBT training. Other treatments may also be considered, such as antidepressant medication. CBT is the first-line treatment recommended for adolescents. What that means is that young people would usually only be prescribed antidepressant medication after they have tried CBT and it hasn't worked, or if their symptoms are very severe. Sometimes both CBT and medication will be recommended. For young people with more mild depression, low-intensity treatments such as group CBT or internet CBT might be recommended in the first instance. There are free, evidence-based internet CBT programmes that are available for young people to use (e.g. MoodGym).

It is important to note that all treatments should be discussed with a trained mental health professional, such as a general practitioner or psychiatrist. The use of antidepressant medication among adolescents should always be considered with caution, and only by those trained in adolescent psychiatry. Treatment choices for adolescent depression are not the same in adults. Hence, it is important to seek specialised help for adolescent depression, such as the local child and adolescent mental health services in your region. Responses to treatment are found to differ greatly, so it is important to keep in regular contact with the healthcare providers to ensure that optimal treatment outcomes are achieved.

Long-term studies have shown that between 60 to 90 per cent of adolescents who have depressive episodes recover from their episode within a year. However, many of these young people (50 to 70 per cent) will go on to experience another depressive episode within five years. This is why seeking treatment is so important – it establishes healthy coping skills and behaviour that can be employed at a later stage if needed. Depression in adolescence is also linked to a range of other mental health disorders in adulthood including anxiety, substance disorders, bipolar disorder and physical health problems. This emphasises the importance of seeking help early in the course of illness, as well as the necessity of prevention interventions. We strongly encourage people not to delay seeking help.

CAN DEPRESSION BE PREVENTED?

Prevention programmes for depression are effective. These usually take the form of CBT, typically delivered to classes of students in the school environment. These programmes teach young people the same skills and strategies they can use to manage their emotions that they would learn in treatment. However, learning about these ways to cope *before* a stressful period can be enormously helpful in reducing the impact and buffering the adolescent against depression, as the young person will have the skills to manage these stressful situations when they arise. Increasingly, CBT programmes are being made available online, which can be less confronting and more engaging to young people, while still communicating the key messages.

WHAT CAN PARENTS DO?

Adolescence is a challenging time for parent–child relations. These strategies can be implemented to help reduce distress:

- When disciplining young people, use positive reinforcement for good behaviour rather than shame and punishment approaches for bad behaviour. Shame and disappointment can make an adolescent feel worthless and inadequate.
- Allow your adolescent to make mistakes. Over-control or over-protection can be perceived as a lack of confidence in their ability to make a decision, and poor trust. This can make them feel less confident, and less likely to turn to you when things are not going so well.

- Accept that your teen will make different choices from you, and don't punish them for that difference. Helping them learn to accept themselves is key to good mental health.
- If you believe your child may be depressed, create a safe space where you can ask them how they are feeling. This needs to be the right location (when it is calm and private) and ensure you have enough time so that you can listen patiently to their concerns. Even if you don't feel that the problem is 'real', remember that it feels very real to them.
- Keep the lines of communication open, even if your teen seems to want to withdraw.
- Avoid telling your teen what to do.
- If there is a close friend or family member, like an older sibling or aunt/uncle, who your teen is close to, you may wish to suggest that your child talks about their concerns with him or her. Sometimes it can be easier for young people to talk to someone other than a parent.
- If you feel overwhelmed or unable to reach out to your child, or you continue to be concerned, seek help from a qualified professional.
- Encourage your child to be active, as physical exercise appears to improve depressive symptoms, as does having good levels of social support and interaction with friends.

TAKE-HOME MESSAGES FOR PARENTS

- If you think your child might be experiencing depression, be supportive but seek professional help. Visiting your doctor is the best place to start.
- Getting in early is critical so don't hesitate, take it seriously.
- Talk to your teenager about how they are feeling.
- Let your child know that you love them and are there for them.
- Create an environment at home where family members are open about their emotions – this will encourage your teen to speak up if they need to.

- Do not be afraid to talk about depression and mental illness with your child.

TAKE-HOME MESSAGES FOR TEACHERS AND SCHOOL COUNSELLORS/YOUTH WORKERS

- If you notice a significant change in the behaviour and emotion of a young person, talk to them about it.
- Create a caring and compassionate school culture by encouraging staff, students and parents to talk about mental health.
- Focusing on the whole young person (not just their academic performance) will help them to be balanced.
- Implementing prevention programmes in the school environment can reduce the risk of depression.

Authors' biographies

Dr Bridianne O'Dea is a mental health researcher at the Black Dog Institute. Her research areas include adolescent mental health, online interventions for depression and anxiety, and social media for suicide prevention. Dr O'Dea is interested in improving mental health through technology.

Dr Aliza Werner-Seidler is a clinical psychologist and mental health researcher at the Black Dog Institute. She conducts clinical research into the prevention and treatment of depression and anxiety in youth with a focus on using technology to develop novel interventions for psychological disorders.

www.blackdoginstitute.org.au

See also:

Chapter 4: Anxiety in Young People
Chapter 18: What is Resilience and How to Do It
Chapter 20: Using Positive Psychology
Chapter 21: Food, Mood and Mental Health

Recommended websites:

Mental Health Foundation: www.mentalhealth.org.uk/a-to-z/despair

NHS: www.nhs.uk/conditions/clinical-depression

Mind: www.mind.org.uk

YoungMinds: youngminds.org.uk

Rethink Mental Illness: www.rethink.org

MoodGym: moodgym.com.au

British Association for Behavioural and Cognitive Psychotherapies: babcp.com

Further resources:

Childline:

    Helpline: 0800 1111

Samaritans:

    Helpline: 116 123

Further reading:

Cairns, KE, Yap, MBH, Pilkington, PD & Jorm, AF 2014, 'Risk and Protective factors for depression that adolescents can modify: A systematic review and meta-analysis of longitudinal studies', *Journal of Affective Disorders*, vol. 169, pp 61–75.

Carter, T, Morres ID, Meade O & Callaghan P 2016, 'The effect of exercise on depressive symptoms in adolescents: A systematic review and meta-analysis', *Journal of the American Academy of Child and Adolescent Psychiatry,* vol. 55, no. 7, pp 580–590.

Cipriani, A, Zhou, X, Giovane, CD, Hetrick, SE, Qin, B, Whittington, C, Coghill, D, Zhang, Y, Hazell, P & Leucht, S et al 2016, 'Comparative efficacy and tolerability of antidepressants for major depressive disorder in children and adolescents: a network meta-analysis', *The Lancet*, vol. 388, no. 10047, pp 881–890.

Ellis, RER, Seal, ML, Simmons, JG, Whittle, S, Schwartz, OS, Byrne, ML & Allen, NB 2016, 'Longitudinal trajectories of depression symptoms in adolescence: psychosocial risk factors and outcomes', *Child Psychiatry and Human Development*.

Hetrick, SE, Cox, GR, Witt, KG, Bir, KK & Merry, SN 2016, 'Evidence-based psychological interventions for preventing depression in children and adolescents', *Cochrane Database of Systematic Reviews*.

Kessler, RC, Berglund, P, Demler, O, Jin, R, Koretz, D, Merikangas, KR, Rush, AJ, Walters, EE & Wang, PS 2003, 'The epidemiology of major depressive disorder: results from the National Comorbidity Survey Replication (NCS-R)'.

McLeod, GFH, Horwood, LJ & Fergusson DM 2016, 'Adolescent depression, adult mental health and psychosocial outcomes at 30 and 35 years', *Psychological Medicine*, vol. 46, no. 7, pp 1401–1412.

O'Dea, B, Calear, AL & Perry, Y, 'Is e-health the answer to gaps in adolescent mental health service delivery?' *Current Opinion in Psychiatry*, vol. 28, no. 1, pp 336–342.

Rueger, SY, Malecki, CK, Pyun, Y, Aycock, C & Coyle, S 2016, 'A meta-analytic review of the association between perceived social support and depression in childhood and adolescence', *Psychological Bulletin*, vol. 142, no. 10, pp 1014–1067.

Salk RH, Petersen J, Abramson LY & Hyde JS 2016, 'The contemporary face of gender differences and similarities in depression throughout adolescence: Development and chronicity', *Journal of Affective Disorders*, vol.205, no. 15, pp 28–35.

Thapar, A, Collishaw, S, Pine, DS & Thapar, AK 2012, 'Depression in adolescence', *The Lancet*, vol. 379, no. 9820, pp 1056–1067.

Werner-Seidler A, Perry Y, Calear A, Newby J & Christensen H 2017, 'School-based depression and anxiety prevention programs for young people: A systematic review and meta-analysis', *Clinical Psychology*, vol. 51, pp 30–47.

For more online resources visit:
generationnext.com.au/handbook

6. UNDERSTANDING SELF-HARM

Dr Claire Kelly

Non-suicidal self-injury is a dysfunctional coping strategy that is often used by young people at times of great distress, and often indicates an underlying mental health problem. This chapter describes the problem and offers advice on how to assist a young person who is engaging in this behaviour.

INTRODUCTION

Non-suicidal self-injury is a maladaptive coping strategy that is sometimes used by young people at times of great distress, and often indicates an underlying mental health problem. The term self-harm is more familiar to many people, and encompasses a broad range of behaviours that are harmful. Non-suicidal self-injury can be more narrowly defined as physical injury that a person inflicts on themselves deliberately as a way of coping with painful and overwhelming feelings.

This chapter will give an overview of the scope and importance of the problem, and then focus on how to provide mental health first aid to a young person who has been engaging in self-injury.

While non-suicidal self-injury affects people of all ages, it is most prevalent in young people. The Australian National Epidemiological Study of Self-Injury (ANESSI) found that among young people aged ten to seventeen, 2 per cent had engaged in self-injury in the last four weeks and 12 per cent at some point in their lifetime.[1] The behaviour was found to be slightly more common in young women than young men.

The median age of onset is just over seventeen years, meaning half of all people who will ever engage in non-suicidal self-injury have done so for the first time by that age. The behaviour is most common in 18- to 24-year-olds. This means that adolescence is the prime time to intervene, in order to find other coping strategies and prevent the behaviour from becoming entrenched.

Non-suicidal self-injury is not a new phenomenon; however, awareness has increased significantly in recent years, and it is probably becoming more prevalent. This makes it a public health issue that is relevant to all adults who work with young people, where the behaviour is most likely to present. It is also an important issue for parents, who are in a prime position to notice the signs of the behaviours and act to engage their children with the professional help that may be required to treat any underlying mental health problems and assist in recovery.

Self-injury is usually associated with mental illness. In the ANESSI study, among participants eighteen years and over, people who engaged in self-injury were more likely to have had a formal diagnosis of depression (6.6 times more likely), an anxiety disorder (5.6 times more likely), attention deficit hyperactivity disorder (ADHD, 8.9 times more likely) or post-traumatic stress disorder (PTSD, 4 times more likely) at some time in their life. Among adolescents, who are less likely to have received mental health treatment, it was highly correlated with a diagnosis of depression (almost 40 times more likely).[2] Many people with mental illnesses never seek help or receive a diagnosis, so the true figures may be much higher.

People who engage in non-suicidal self-injury are also more likely to use substances of all kinds (including tobacco) and more likely to use alcohol to deliberately get drunk. Only data collected from the same people over many years would enable researchers to understand the relationship (whether a history of self-injury increases the chances of substance misuse, or whether substance misuse increases the risk of self-injury). However, it may be that people who have trouble managing their emotions are more likely to use external coping strategies to change the way they feel, including both self-injury and substance use. This is another reason to help a young person to find positive coping strategies as early as possible.

Finally, non-suicidal self-injury is an important risk factor for suicide and attempted suicide.[3] This means that responding to self-injury with kindness and empathy, and seeking help for the underlying mental health problems, is both important and urgent to reduce the risk. Responding with anger, or ignoring the behaviour as attention-seeking, may increase the risk.

DEFINITIONS

Non-suicidal self-injury: deliberately causing harm to oneself without intent to die.

Self-harm: any action or behaviour that causes oneself harm, including non-suicidal self-injury, suicide attempts, substance misuse and risk-taking behaviour.

Mental illness: a diagnosable illness that causes major changes in thinking, feeling and behaviour, and interferes with daily functioning.

Mental health problem: an umbrella term that refers to mental illnesses as well as developing problems, where the symptoms might not yet be severe enough, frequent enough, or consistent enough to warrant a diagnosis of mental illness.

Mental health first aid: the help given to a person who is developing a mental health problem, experiencing a worsening of an existing mental health problem, or in a mental health crisis. The help is given until appropriate professional help has been received, or the crisis has resolved.

WHY DO PEOPLE INJURE THEMSELVES?

There are many reasons why people injure themselves. The most common are:

- To manage painful feelings (57 per cent).
- To punish oneself (25 per cent).
- To communicate with others (6 per cent).

Less than 3 per cent cited their reason as combatting suicidal thoughts, seeking a rush or high, or to deliberately scar themselves.

The overall theme is that the current emotional state is unbearable, and self-injury can change the state enough to make it bearable for a while.

Self-injury is rarely used as a means of 'seeking attention', due to the intense shame most people feel about their wounds and scars. However, for some people displaying injuries may be the only language they have which might communicate to others that they are in need of help. Rather than viewing this behaviour as 'attention-seeking', it's more helpful to view it as 'attention *needing*'.

THE MENTAL HEALTH FIRST AID GUIDELINES

The advice offered in this chapter comes from research conducted with an international panel of experts on non-suicidal self-injury.[4] The panel included professional experts (both clinicians and researchers) and those with personal experience of non-suicidal self-injury (both individuals and caregivers), from Australia, Canada, New Zealand, the UK and the USA. Participants were presented with statements sourced from both medical and lay literature, and asked to rate their suitability for inclusion in the guidelines. This method makes it possible to draw from a broad knowledge base and provide the best possible advice.

The advice also draws from guidelines developed for communicating with adolescents about difficult and sensitive topics. These guidelines were developed in the same way.

The full text of the of guidelines is available from the Mental Health First Aid website: www.mhfa.com.au.

HOW DO PEOPLE INJURE THEMSELVES?

There are many forms of non-suicidal self-injury. However, in the ANESSI study the most common methods were found to be cutting (41 per cent) or scratching (40 per cent) the skin, deliberately hitting a body part against a hard surface (37 per cent), punching or otherwise hitting self (34 per cent), biting and burning (both 15 per cent). Cutting and scratching are both more common in women than men and both types of hitting are more common in men. It is useful to keep this in mind when assisting a young man who could easily be dismissed as angry or aggressive; punching a wall when angry, frustrated and overwhelmed may be better interpreted as trying to manage overwhelming emotions, and young men who do this may need support, rather than a disciplinary response.

Self-injury ranges in severity. A cut may be medically superficial and draw very little blood, or it may be deep enough to expose fat, muscle or even bone. Hitting can result in mild bruising or broken bones. No relationship has been proven between the severity of the injury and the severity of the emotional distress, so it's important not to dismiss medically superficial injury as not warranting concern.

WHAT SHOULD I DO IF I SUSPECT SOMEONE IS SELF-INJURING?

If you suspect that a young person you care about has been injuring themselves, you need to discuss it with them. Before you approach them, acknowledge and deal with your own feelings about the behaviour so these don't get in the way. If you feel you are unable to talk to the person who is self-injuring, try to find someone else who can talk to them.

Choose a private place for the conversation. Directly express your concerns that the young person may be injuring themselves. Ask about self-injury in a way that makes it clear that you understand a bit about the subject, e.g. 'Sometimes, when people are in a lot of emotional pain, they injure themselves on purpose. Is that how your injury happened?' Do not demand to talk about things the person is not ready to discuss.

HOW CAN I TELL IF SOMEONE HAS BEEN INJURING THEMSELVES?

It can be difficult to know for sure if a young person has been injuring themselves, as there is often a lot of shame around both injuries and scars, leading the young person to work hard to keep evidence concealed. There are some signs worth keeping in mind, though.

- **Frequent suspicious injuries**, particularly if they are similar each time, e.g. scratches on the same part of the arm. If you don't see such injuries, you might notice the young person avoids being touched or bumped even through clothing where they are injured.
- **Long sleeves or trousers in hot weather**, where this is unusual for the person. Be aware, though, that some people injure their upper thighs, stomach, breasts or other areas that would routinely be covered up.
- If you live with the young person, you may notice **first aid supplies being used more quickly than usual**, or blood on clothing or bedsheets.

It's important to listen to your own suspicions, though. If you believe that a young person you care about might be injuring themselves, you should ask them in a way that shows you care and want to help, that you have empathy, and that you understand a little bit about non-suicidal self-injury. This will hopefully make it easier for them to have a frank conversation with you.

WHAT SHOULD I DO IF I FIND SOMEONE INJURING THEMSELVES?

If you witness someone injuring themselves, intervene in a supportive and non-judgemental way. Although it is natural to feel upset, helpless and even angry, try to remain calm and avoid expressions of shock or anger. Tell the person that you are concerned about them and ask whether you can do anything to alleviate the distress. Ask if medical attention is needed.

When is emergency medical attention needed?

Avoid overreacting; medical attention is only required if the injury is severe. Contact emergency services if a wound or injury is serious. Any cut that is gaping requires medical attention, as it may need stitches or another medical closure. Any burn that is two centimetres or larger in diameter, and any burn on the hands, feet or face requires medical attention.

If the young person has harmed themselves by taking an overdose of medication or consuming poison, call an ambulance, as the risk of death or serious harm is high. Deliberate overdose is more frequently intended to result in death, but is sometimes a form of self-injury. Regardless of a person's intentions, emergency help must be sought.

If you take or accompany a young person to hospital, ask for a mental health assessment and be an advocate and supporter. There is stigma about self-injury that can result in a young person being treated poorly by medical professionals who do not have adequate understanding of mental illness and think that kindness and empathy may reinforce the behaviour.

How should I talk with a young person who has been engaging in self-injury?

Keep in mind that 'stopping self-injury' should not be the focus of the conversation. Instead, look at what can be done to make the young person's life more manageable, or their environment less distressing. Understand that self-injury won't stop overnight, and the young person will need time to recover and learn healthy coping mechanisms.

Behave in a supportive and non-judgemental way. Understand that self-injury makes the person's life easier and accept their reasons for doing it. Be supportive without being permissive of the behaviour. Be aware of what your body language is communicating about your attitudes.

Use a calm voice when talking to the person. Avoid expressing anger or a desire to punish the person for self-injuring. Be comfortable with silence, allowing the person time to process what has been talked about. Be prepared for the expression of intense emotions.

WHAT SHOULD I SAY?

Express concern and actively listen

Tell the young person that you want to help. Ask questions about their self-injury, but avoid pressuring them to talk about it. Reflect what the person is saying by acknowledging their experience as they are describing it. See box titled 'Communicating with care and empathy'.

Try to talk 'with' them, not 'at' them. Do not do all of the talking. It is best to let the young person set the pace and style of your conversation, if they are able to. After speaking, be patient and allow plenty of time for the young person to collect their thoughts, reflect on their feelings and decide what to say next. Don't be afraid to ask open, honest questions without expressing judgement. Ask the adolescent about their experiences and how they feel about them, rather than make your own interpretation.

Give support and reassurance

Express empathy for how the person is feeling. Endorse the person's emotions by explaining that these emotions are appropriate and valid.

Let them know they are not alone and that you are there to support them. Work collaboratively with the person in finding solutions (i.e. by finding out what they want to happen, and discussing any possible actions with them).

Reassure the person that there are sources of help and support available. Tell the person that you want to help, and let them know the ways in which you are willing to help them.

Don't promise the person that you will keep their self-injury a secret. If you need to tell somebody about the person's self-injury to keep them safe, speak to them about this first. Avoid gossiping or talking to others about it without their permission.

Consider your body language

Communicating with care and empathy is not just about what you say, but how you say it. Consider your body language: are you standing or sitting in a way that makes you tower over the young person? Arms crossed over your body or hands on your hips can communicate anger, even if you don't feel angry.

It is good to find a place where you can both sit comfortably, with open posture, angled towards each other. Maintain comfortable eye contact and allow for periods of silence.

COMMUNICATING WITH CARE AND EMPATHY

Self-injury is a very private thing and is hard to talk about. You should avoid expressing a strong emotional response of anger, fear, revulsion or frustration. Finding caring and non-judgemental ways to talk about injury is important. Think about some specific sentences you might use, or questions you might ask, before you approach the young person.

Use 'I' statements.
DON'T say: 'You really worry me when you do these things.'
This 'you' statement is likely to trigger defensiveness, and blames the young person for your own emotional state.
DO say: 'I am really worried about you.'
This 'I' statement allows you to own your behaviour and emotions – the worry – without implying it is what the young person set out to do.

Focus on the young person's need to cope, rather than their behaviour.

DON'T say: 'You have to stop this. It's dangerous and you will end up with scars.'

It takes time to find new coping strategies, and it is not an easy thing to do. If the young person had a better coping strategy available, which worked as well as self-injury does, they would use that instead. This sort of tone may also trigger the young person's need to punish themselves, as it implies that they are doing something wrong.

DO say: 'We can get you the help you need to find other ways to cope.'

This shows that you understand that self-injury is a coping strategy and that just stopping is not a viable option, until there are other strategies in place.

If the person shows you their injuries, don't accuse them of attention-seeking.

DON'T say: 'You're manipulative/passive aggressive/just after attention.'

If the person does show you their injuries, this might be their way of asking for help. Attention-seeking should not be regarded as negatively as it is in the community. It might not be the most functional way to ask for help, but the person can be trying to show you just how much pain they are in. This sort of language makes it hard for a person to ask for help again, from you or anyone else.

DO say: 'We can find other ways for you to ask for help.'

Tell the young person that help is available, and that they can ask for and receive help without needing to hurt themselves.

WHAT DO I DO IF THE PERSON IS NOT READY TO TALK?

Respect the young person's right not to talk about their self-injuring. If the person doesn't want to talk right away:

- Let them know that you want to listen to them when they are ready.

- Ask the person what would make them feel safe enough to be able to discuss their feelings.
- Ask if there is someone else they would feel more comfortable talking to.
- Follow up with them in a day or two. Having some time to think about what you have said might motivate them to come back to you, but they may not have the psychological maturity or life skills to approach you. By remaining as approachable as practical, and consistent in your words and actions, you can build a relationship which might make it easier to talk.

Do not force the issue unless the injury is severe. If the person still doesn't want to talk, ask a health professional for advice on what to do.

SEEKING PROFESSIONAL HELP

Self-injury is often a symptom of a mental health problem that can be treated. Encourage the person to seek professional help. Let them remain in control over seeking help as much as possible. Suggest and discuss options for getting help rather than directing the person what to do. Help the person map out a plan of action for seeking help. Talk about how you can help them to seek treatment and who they can talk to, e.g. a mental health service or a mental health professional.

Provide praise for any steps the person takes towards getting professional help. Follow up with the person to check whether they have found professional help that is suitable for them.

You should seek mental health assistance on the person's behalf if:

- The person asks you to.
- The injury is severe or getting more severe, such as cuts getting deeper or bones being broken.
- The self-injurious behaviour is interfering with daily life.
- The person has injured their eyes.
- The person has injured their genitals.
- The person has expressed a desire to die.

If the person is an adolescent, a more directive approach may be needed. Help the young person map out a plan of action for seeking help and offer to go along with them to an appointment.

What if they don't want help?

Keep in mind that not all people who self-injure want to change their behaviour. Even though you can offer support, you are not responsible for the actions or behaviour of someone else, and cannot control what they do. Unless the injury is severe or life-threatening, the person can't be compelled to accept treatment.

This doesn't mean you should give up. Continue to encourage the young person to seek or accept help. Remember that there is probably an underlying mental health problem that makes it even harder to accept help. It can be helpful to consider what other signs of mental health problems are present, and give the person information about these.

For example, if the person is also weepy at times, has had changes in their sleeping or eating patterns, or can't seem to get any enjoyment out of things they used to enjoy, they might be suffering from depression. While you can't make a diagnosis of depression, it's okay to let the person know that you've seen signs that concern you and which might be symptoms of depression. It can be a motivator, if the person knows that help is available and you think they would benefit from talking to a mental health professional about it.

ENCOURAGING ALTERNATIVES TO SELF-INJURY

Encourage the person to seek other ways to relieve their distress. Help the person to use their coping strategies that do not involve self-injuring, and help them to make a plan about what to do when they feel like self-injuring. Suggest some coping strategies and discuss with the person what might be helpful for them.

Encourage the use of any positive coping strategy which helps them to get through the urge to self-injure. Encourage the person to share their feelings with other people, such as a close friend or family member, when they are feeling distressed or have the urge to self-injure. Help the person think of ways to reduce their distress, for example, having a hot bath, listening to loud music, or doing something kind for themselves. Offer the person information materials (e.g. a website or factsheet) about alternatives to self-injury.

ALTERNATIVES TO SELF-INJURY

When trying to stop engaging in non-suicidal self-injury, it can take time to find new ways to cope. While the person is waiting for professional help, or when times are tough, it's good to have a few alternatives to self-injury. The best option is one they come up with themselves; but if the young person is feeling overwhelmed, it can be hard to think of anything. You may wish to discuss some of the options below.

This list is not exhaustive. Suggestions in this list may appeal more to some young people than to others.

Talk to someone

- Encourage the young person to tell a friend or family member how they feel, and why they are upset.
- Encourage the young person to talk to a friend or family member about other things, and see if focusing on something different helps them to cope with the urge to injure.
- If they don't think they can talk to someone they know, encourage them to call a helpline. Childline (for anyone under the age of nineteen in the UK): 0800 1111.

Delay – The urge to injure doesn't last forever.

- Encourage the young person to wait for five minutes, congratulate themselves on that achievement, and then wait five minutes more, or maybe ten. Their level of distress will come down, but it will take time.
- Most young people who injure do so when they are alone, and often in a familiar setting, such as their bedroom or bathroom. Encourage them to go elsewhere and be around people.

Distract – Encourage the young person to do something engrossing, such as:

- Watch a film, especially something that might make them laugh or bring another strong positive emotional response.
- Do some exercise. Exercise boosts brain chemicals such as endorphins and may improve mood.
- Do something creative. Maybe you can find others ways to express negative emotions, such as art, creative writing, making music or dancing.

Do something else – If the young person can figure out what brought on the urge to injure, you may be able to help them to fulfil it in a different way, one that isn't harmful.

- Needing to feel something can be fulfilled by holding ice or touching textures.
- Needing to see blood can be fulfilled by drawing on skin with red ink or paint.
- If the person feels the need to punish themselves, try to help them find a way to be kind to themselves instead, or to forgive themselves.

Discourage the young person from engaging in activities that are harmful or cause pain. This can help to break the association between pain and relief.

IS SELF-INJURY 'CONTAGIOUS'?

School professionals in particular are often concerned that non-suicidal self-injury in one young person may spread to their peers. It's important to keep in mind that while young people may try things they've seen peers do, if self-injury isn't serving a purpose, it won't become a habit or a pattern.

Where a group of young people have developed a pattern of self-injury, it is likely that all or most are experiencing a degree of distress and vulnerability. It might be beneficial to look at ways to support the whole group to find positive coping strategies, and also to support each other.

SOME WORDS OF ADVICE FOR PARENTS

When a young person has a mental health problem, parents can experience a wide range of reactions. It is easy to respond out of fear, disbelief or even anger. However, this is likely to prompt your child to try to hide the behaviour more effectively, and make it harder for them to talk openly with you. Do your best to manage your reactions, and focus on what you can do to reduce your child's distress. Avoid talking about how scars might impact them later on.

CONCLUSION

Non-suicidal self-injury is a serious problem. It can become the primary coping strategy for negative emotions, the injuries and scars provoke stigmatising attitudes from both medical professionals and the public, and engaging in self-injury increases the long-term risk of suicide. However, when viewed as a coping strategy for an underlying problem, offering help becomes less daunting. Depression and anxiety are common underlying mental health problems related to non-suicidal self-injury, and effective treatment is available for both.

Genuine concern and compassion for young people who engage in self-injury can make it easier for them to accept help, or seek it on their own, reducing the long-term problems associated with the behaviour.

The author would like to acknowledge Anna Ross, Anthony Jorm and Betty Kitchener, co-authors of the *Mental health first aid guidelines for non-suicidal self-injury*.

Author biography

Dr Claire Kelly is the manager of youth programmes at Mental Health First Aid Australia. She has been a main contributor to the mental health first aid guidelines projects. Claire has experienced episodes of depression and anxiety since early adolescence, which has been a driver for her work.

www.mhfa.com.au

See also:
Chapter 1: Helping Young People Get Help for Mental Health Problems
Chapter 2: What to do in a Mental Health Crisis
Chapter 4: Anxiety in Young People
Chapter 5: Depression in Young People

Recommended websites:
Mental Health First Aid: www.mhfa.com.au or www.mhfaengland.org
NHS: www.nhs.uk/conditions/self-harm
Harmless: www.harmless.org.uk
National Self Harm Network: www.nshn.co.uk
LifeSIGNS: www.lifesigns.org.uk
Self-injury Support: www.selfinjurysupport.org.uk

Further resources:
Childline:
   Helpline: 0800 1111

Samaritans:
   Helpline: 116 123

Further reading:
Fischer JA, Kelly CM, Kitchener BA & Jorm AF 2013, 'Development of Guidelines for Adults on How to Communicate With Adolescents About Mental Health Problems and Other Sensitive Topics', *Sage Open*, vol. 3, no. 4.

Mental Health First Aid Australia 2014, *Communicating with adolescents: guidelines for adults on how to communicate with adults about mental health problems and other sensitive topics*, Mental Health First Aid Australia, Melbourne.

Mental Health First Aid Australia 2015, *Non-suicidal self-injury: first aid guidelines*, Mental Health First Aid Australia, Melbourne.

 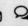

7. SUICIDE AND ATTEMPTED SUICIDE

Dr Claire Kelly

Suicide is the most common cause of death among young people, accounting for a third of deaths among sixteen to twenty-four-year-olds. Suicide is often preventable, if people are able to recognise the signs and act quickly.

INTRODUCTION

Suicide is the most common cause of death among people under forty-five, and it accounts for a third of deaths among sixteen to twenty-four-year-olds. Young people under twenty-five report very high rates of suicidality and suicide attempts, most of which go unreported to health professionals. Suicide is often preventable, if people are able to recognise the signs and act quickly. Mental health first aid guidelines have been developed to help people respond and intervene to prevent suicide and get young people the help they need.

Suicide in young people is a major concern in many countries. This is because suicide is the biggest killer of adolescents and young adults. The second most common cause of death in this age group is motor vehicle injuries, accounting for 14 per cent of deaths. Although deaths from motor vehicle injuries have declined significantly in recent years, successes in reducing the death rate from suicide has tapered off, and the rate appears to be climbing again. In Australia in 2015, the Australian Bureau of Statistics reports there were 3027 suicides in all age groups, the culmination of a steady increase over the last several years, representing an increase of 43 per cent over the 2118 deaths from suicide in 2006. The suicide rate among young people aged sixteen to twenty-four increased by 30 per cent over the same period.

THREE BIG MYTHS

There are a lot of myths about suicide that are prevalent in the community. Here are three big ones you might have heard, and what to say if you encounter them.

Myth: Talking about suicide will put the idea into people's heads.
Fact: This isn't true. The evidence tells us that a person who has the opportunity to talk about their suicidal thoughts is less likely to act on them. Conversely, if the person isn't having thoughts of suicide, you have communicated strongly to them that you are a person who is willing to talk about it in the future.

Myth: People who talk about suicide don't do it.
Fact: This isn't true. Most people who die by suicide try to tell someone about their thoughts. Often it's not taken seriously, or dismissed as a 'cry for help'. Think about this for a minute: if someone has had an accident and broken a bone, and is literally crying for help, we don't dismiss that. Why dismiss someone who is talking about suicide?

Myth: If the person is planning to die by taking pills, they are not really serious.
Fact: Self-poisoning is the second most common method of suicide after hanging, and the most common method of suicide attempt that does not result in death. Compared to someone who uses hanging, a person who has taken an overdose has a better chance of being interrupted by someone who can get them help, changing their mind and seeking help for themselves, or misjudging the dose and surviving by accident. It doesn't mean they weren't serious.

Although statistics are important, particularly when we want to monitor for change, they can't adequately describe the human cost of suicide. For every young person who ends their life, there are future possibilities that abruptly cease to be. There are family members and friends who feel the loss, and ripples felt across the whole community.

For every death by suicide, there are many suicide attempts that do not result in death. Young people have a higher rate of suicidal thoughts and behaviours than other age groups. Recent Australian research found that 7.5 per cent of adolescents aged twelve to seventeen had thoughts of suicide each year, and 2.4 per cent had made a suicide attempt.[1] Other Australian research revealed that among sixteen to twenty-four-year-olds, 3.4 per cent had serious thoughts of suicide and 1.1 per cent had made a suicide attempt in the last twelve months.[2] Even suicide attempts that do not result in death can have serious consequences such as organ damage, lasting injuries and permanent disability, as well as emotional consequences, damage to family and social relationships, and even to a person's reputation.

THE SPECTRUM OF SUICIDE REDUCTION ACTIVITIES

Suicide reduction activities take many forms. As 87 per cent of people who die by suicide have a mental illness, efforts to improve mental health in the community through education and early intervention count towards these efforts. However, I am going to focus here on those activities that target suicide and suicidal behaviour directly, grouped loosely into *universal prevention, targeted prevention* and *suicide intervention*.

Universal prevention activities are those that target the entire population. This ranges from services provided to anyone who wishes to use them (such as Samaritans) through to advertising public health messages about seeking help if you are having thoughts of suicide.

Targeted prevention activities focus on groups at high risk of suicide. For example, efforts in recent years have encouraged boys and men to talk about depression, hopefully enabling early intervention for depression, and therefore reducing the risk of suicide. Other groups at risk in Australia include young lesbian, gay, bisexual, transgender, intersex, and queer and questioning (LGBTIQ) people, so specific outreach services have been created with those communities in mind. Suicide prevention activities are important. However, they won't reach everyone. Someone who is in few or no specific high-risk groups can still be at risk of suicide.

Suicide first aid and *suicide intervention* focus on individuals. These activities provide education for health professionals and the public to identify warning signs in individuals and act to keep them safe. They are provided in a number of different settings and vary a little from state to state. Some examples will be provided at the end of this chapter.

The focus of this chapter will be on mental health first aid for suicidal thoughts and behaviours. Mental health first aid is the help given to a person who is developing a mental health problem, experiencing a worsening of an existing mental health problem, or in a mental health crisis. The help is given until appropriate professional help has been received, or the crisis has resolved.

MENTAL HEALTH FIRST AID FOR SUICIDAL THOUGHTS AND BEHAVIOURS

WHERE DID THESE GUIDELINES COME FROM?

The content of these guidelines was developed via the Delphi methodology.[3] In brief, this is a method for reaching consensus within and between groups of experts. This study involved two groups of experts: professionals (including researchers and clinicians) and those with lived experience (including people who had experienced thoughts of suicide or attempted suicide, and people who were caregivers for those with direct lived experience, who were now acting in some kind of advocacy role in the community). They were presented with a long list of statements that had been made in the medical and lay literature and asked to rate how important each was as a guideline for a member of the public with no clinical training. Statements rated as *important* or *essential* by 80 per cent or more of both panels were included in the final guidelines.

The guidelines are not exhaustive. They are designed to be a set of actions that will help most people, most of the time. The relationship between the person at risk of suicide and the first aider needs to be taken into consideration, and it's important that the first aider is flexible and prepared to seek professional help if they feel they can't manage on their own.

Suicide can be prevented. Most suicidal people do not want to die. They simply do not want to live with the pain. Openly talking about suicidal thoughts and feelings can save a life. Do not underestimate your abilities to help a suicidal young person.

REASONS WHY A PERSON MIGHT HAVE THOUGHTS ABOUT SUICIDE

The main reasons people give for attempting suicide are:

- Needing to escape or relieve unmanageable emotions and thoughts. The person wants relief from unbearable emotional pain, feels their situation is hopeless, feels worthless and believes that other people would be better off without them.
- Desire to communicate with or influence another individual. The person wants to communicate how they feel to other people, change how other people treat them or get help.

FACTORS ASSOCIATED WITH A HIGHER RISK OF SUICIDE

People are at greater risk of suicide if they have:

- a mental illness.
- poor physical health or disabilities.
- attempted suicide or harmed themselves in the past.

- had bad things happen recently, particularly with relationships or their health.
- been physically or sexually abused as a child.
- been recently exposed to suicide by someone else, e.g. recent loss of a family member or friend to suicide.

Suicide is also more common in certain groups, including males, Indigenous people, the unemployed, prisoners, and gay, lesbian and bisexual people.

HOW CAN I TELL IF SOMEONE IS FEELING SUICIDAL?

It is important that you know the warning signs and risk factors for suicide, and the reasons why a person might have thoughts of suicide.

SIGNS A PERSON MAY BE SUICIDAL CAN INCLUDE:

- Threatening to hurt or kill themselves.
- Looking for ways to kill themselves: seeking access to pills, weapons, or other means.
- Talking or writing about death, dying or suicide.
- Hopelessness.
- Rage, anger, seeking revenge.
- Acting recklessly or engaging in risky activities, seemingly without thinking.
- Feeling trapped, like there's no way out.
- Increasing alcohol and drug use.
- Withdrawing from friends, family or society.
- Anxiety, agitation, unable to sleep or sleeping all the time.
- Dramatic changes in mood.
- No reason for living, no sense of purpose in life.

Some people will show several of these signs, and others will show signs that are not on this list. It's important that you don't ignore your own suspicions, especially when helping a young person you know well.

SIGNS A SCHOOL PROFESSIONAL MIGHT NOTICE

Talking or writing about death, dying or suicide might be something explicitly spoken, or it might be more subtle. Art and other creative works, including writing, film-making and theatre, could give clues to the young person's state of mind. When choosing a topic for an essay, a student might choose suicide or mental illness to write about.

These are only clues. A young person who has shifted from bright colours and happy scenes to death imagery might simply be exploring the possibilities of different styles. It is still important to investigate through the use of direct questioning.

If you are concerned the person may be at risk of suicide, you need to approach them and have a conversation about your concerns.

Preparing yourself to approach the person

Be aware of your own attitudes about suicide and how these could affect your ability to help, e.g. a belief that suicide is wrong or that young people only talk about suicide to get attention. Be aware that the young person might have beliefs and attitudes about suicide that differ from your own, especially if they are from a different cultural or religious background.

Don't let that put you off trying to help, though. It is more important to genuinely want to help than to be of the same age, gender or cultural background as the person.

If you feel unable to ask the young person about suicidal thoughts, find someone else who can.

If you think a young person is considering suicide, you need to act quickly. Even if you only have a mild suspicion that the person is having suicidal thoughts, you should still approach them.

Tell them that you care and want to help. Tell them your concerns about them, describing behaviours that have caused you to be concerned about suicide. For example:

- 'You've seemed unhappy in the last few weeks, and now I see that you've cancelled the appointment we had scheduled to discuss university options. Sometimes when people have lost sight of the future, it's because they're not planning to be here for it.'
- 'I'm concerned about you, because you've stopped seeing your counsellor, and now you've told me you gave away your grandmother's necklace to a friend. I know that it was very important to you.'

However, understand that the person may not want to talk to you. In this instance, you should offer to help them find someone else to talk to. Also, if you are unable to make a connection with the person, help them to find someone else to talk to.

Asking about thoughts of suicide

Anyone could have thoughts of suicide. If you think someone might be having suicidal thoughts, you should ask that person directly. Unless someone tells you, the only way to know if they are thinking about suicide is to ask.

For example, you could ask:

- 'Are you having thoughts of suicide?' *or*
- 'Are you thinking about killing yourself?'

While it is more important to ask the question directly than to be concerned about the exact wording, you should not ask about suicide in leading or judgemental ways, e.g. 'You're not thinking of doing anything stupid, are you?'

Sometimes people are reluctant to ask directly about suicide because they think they will put the idea in the person's head. This is not true. Similarly, if a person is suicidal, asking them about suicidal thoughts will not increase the risk that they will act on these. Instead, asking the person about suicidal thoughts will allow them the chance to talk about their problems and show them that somebody cares.

Although it is common to feel panic or shock when someone tells you about their thoughts of suicide, it is important to avoid expressing negative reactions. Do your best to appear calm, confident and empathetic in the face of the suicide crisis, as this may have a reassuring effect for the suicidal person.

HOW SHOULD I TALK TO A YOUNG PERSON WHO IS SUICIDAL?

It is more important to be genuinely caring than to say 'all the right things'. Be supportive and understanding, and listen with undivided attention. Suicidal thoughts are often a plea for help and a desperate attempt to escape from problems and distressing feelings. *A plea for help should not be regarded as a person being 'just after attention'.* Remember that everyone needs attention at times, and people who are distressed are more in need.

Ask the young person what they are thinking and feeling. Reassure them that you want to hear whatever they have to say. Allow them to talk about these thoughts and feelings, and their reasons for wanting to die, and acknowledge these. Let the suicidal person know it is okay to talk about things that might be painful, even if it is hard. Allow them to express their feelings, e.g. allow them to cry, express anger, or scream. They may feel relief at being able to do so. Thank the suicidal person for sharing their feelings with you and acknowledge the courage this takes.

LISTENING TIPS

- Be patient and calm while the suicidal person is talking about their feelings.
- Listen to the suicidal person without expressing judgement, accepting what they are saying without agreeing or disagreeing with their behaviour or point of view.
- Ask open-ended questions (i.e. questions that cannot be simply answered with 'yes' or 'no') to find out more about the suicidal thoughts and feelings and the problems behind these.

- Show you are listening by summarising what the suicidal person is saying.
- Clarify important points with the person to make sure they are fully understood.
- Express empathy for the suicidal person.

WHAT YOU SHOULD NOT DO WHEN TALKING TO A SUICIDAL PERSON

- Do not argue or debate with the person about their thoughts of suicide.
- Do not discuss with the person whether suicide is right or wrong.
- Do not use guilt or threats to prevent suicide (e.g. do not tell the person they will go to hell or ruin other people's lives if they die by suicide).
- Do not minimise the suicidal person's problems.
- Do not give glib 'reassurance' such as 'don't worry', 'cheer up', 'you have everything going for you' or 'everything will be all right'.
- Do not interrupt with stories of your own.
- Do not communicate a lack of interest or negative attitude through your body language.
- Do not 'call their bluff' (dare or tell the suicidal person to 'just do it').
- Do not attempt to give the suicidal person a diagnosis of a mental illness.

LANGUAGE AND SUICIDE

Do not avoid using the word 'suicide'. It is important to discuss the issue directly without dread or expressing negative judgement. When we try to soften language around suicide, we can communicate the idea that it's not okay to talk about it, or we can avoid frank conversations about it. For example, when we use a term like 'hurting yourself' instead of suicide, a young person might think we are talking about non-suicidal self-injury.

It's important to use appropriate language that doesn't promote stigma.

- Don't say 'commit suicide'. This language implies that suicide is a crime or a sin.
- Don't refer to a suicide attempt as 'successful' or 'unsuccessful'. This implies that dying is the better outcome.
- Don't refer to a suicide attempt as having 'failed'. Again, this makes it sound as if death would have been a success. It can also lead a young person to think that they should try again and succeed this time.

HOW CAN I TELL HOW URGENT THE SITUATION IS?

Take all thoughts of suicide seriously and take action. Do not dismiss the person's thoughts as 'attention-seeking' or a 'cry for help'. Determine the urgency of taking action based on recognition of suicide warning signs.

Ask the suicidal person about issues that affect their immediate safety:

- Whether they have a plan for suicide.
- How they intend to suicide, i.e. ask them direct questions about how and where they intend to suicide.
- Whether they have decided when they will carry out their plan.
- Whether they have already taken steps to secure the means to end their life.
- Whether they have been using drugs or alcohol. Intoxication can increase the risk of a person acting on suicidal thoughts.
- Whether they have ever attempted or planned suicide in the past.

If the suicidal person says they are hearing voices, ask what the voices are telling them. This is important in case the voices are relevant to their current suicidal thoughts.

It is also useful to find out what supports are available to the person:

- Whether they have told anyone about how they are feeling.
- Whether there have been changes in their employment, social life or family.
- Whether they have received treatment for mental health problems or are taking any medication.

Be aware that those at the highest risk for acting on thoughts of suicide in the near future are those who have a specific suicide plan, the means to carry out the plan, a time set for doing it, and an intention to do it. However, the lack of a plan for suicide is not sufficient to ensure safety.

HOW CAN I KEEP THE PERSON SAFE?

A young person who is suicidal should not be left on their own. If you think there is an immediate risk of the person acting on suicidal thoughts, act quickly, even if you are unsure. If possible, work together with the young person to ensure their safety, rather than taking control.

Tell the young person that suicidal thoughts need not be acted on, and reassure them that there are solutions to problems or ways of coping other than suicide. This is not the same as trying to solve the young person's problems directly. For example, a young person who was being bullied, and had begun to think of suicide as an escape, might benefit from learning about what can be done to stop the bullying, but probably won't be persuaded by someone saying that they will somehow make it go away.

When talking to the suicidal young person, focus on the things that will keep them safe for now, rather than the things that put them at risk, e.g. focus on getting professional help, rather than talking about the bullying they have experienced. To help keep them safe, work together to develop a safety plan.

Although you can offer support, you are not responsible for the actions or behaviours of someone else, and cannot control what they might decide to do.

SAFETY PLAN

A safety plan is an agreement between the suicidal person and the first aider that involves actions to keep the person safe. The safety plan should:

- Focus on what the suicidal person should do rather than what they shouldn't.
- Be clear, outlining what will be done, who will be doing it, and when it will be carried out.
- Specify a length of time that will be easy for the suicidal person to cope with, so that they can feel able to fulfil the agreement and have a sense of achievement.
- Include contact numbers that the person agrees to call if they are feeling suicidal, e.g. the person's doctor or mental health care professional, a suicide helpline or twenty-four-hour crisis line, friends and family members who will help in an emergency.

WHAT ABOUT PROFESSIONAL HELP?

Encourage the young person to get appropriate professional help as soon as possible, and be prepared to be directive if necessary. If you are not a family member, make sure someone close to them is aware of the situation, e.g. a close friend or family member, or someone who can take responsibility for them. If they refuse to seek professional help, you will need to seek it on their behalf. While it is best to have the young person's cooperation, their safety takes priority.

If a young person believes that involving their parents will endanger them, seek the advice of a mental health professional, or the headteacher if you are a school professional.

Find out information about the resources and services available for a young person who is considering suicide, including local services that can assist in response to people at risk of suicide. Provide this information to the young person and discuss help-seeking options with them. If they don't want to talk to someone face to face, encourage them to contact a telephone counselling line such as Childline.

Don't assume that the young person will get better without help or that they will seek help on their own. People who are feeling suicidal often don't ask for help for many reasons, including stigma, shame and a belief that their situation is hopeless and that nothing can help. Young people in particular often don't seek help at all, unless someone they trust encourages them to do so and helps them.

For people at more urgent risk, additional action may be needed to facilitate professional help seeking. Seek help if:

- You do not believe the young person can stay safe.
- The young person has a specific suicide plan.
- The young person has the means to carry out a plan (e.g. pills) and will not give them up.

It is better if the young person will cooperate on choosing who to seek help from. However, once again, safety must take priority. Seek the advice of a mental health professional or crisis assessment team if the young person can't identify someone they are willing to talk to.

If the young person has a weapon, contact the police. When contacting the police, inform them that the person is suicidal to help them respond appropriately. Make sure you do not put yourself in any danger. However, remember that it is very rare for a person who is considering suicide to instead hurt someone else.

Be prepared for the suicidal young person to possibly express anger and feel betrayed by your attempt to prevent their suicide or assist them in getting professional help. Try not to take personally any hurtful actions or words.

THE PERSON I AM TRYING TO HELP HAS INJURED THEMSELVES, BUT SAYS THEY ARE NOT SUICIDAL. WHAT SHOULD I DO?

Some people injure themselves for reasons other than suicide. This may be to relieve unbearable anguish, to stop feeling numb, or other reasons. This can be distressing to see. The chapter titled *'Understanding Self-harm'* can help you to understand and assist if this is occurring.

ADVICE TO PARENTS

If your child is having thoughts of suicide, you may experience a range of reactions, including guilt that you have somehow failed them, and anger that they could consider something so drastic when you have provided and sacrificed for them. All emotional responses are valid; however, some are not helpful.

Try to maintain your focus on what your child is experiencing. If you react in a way that stops them from talking to you, it can be hard to make progress. Instead, tell them that they have been courageous in talking to you about what is happening for them and, later on, talk to someone you trust about how you are feeling.

WHAT IF THE PERSON WANTS ME TO PROMISE NOT TO TELL ANYONE ELSE?

You must never agree to keep a plan for suicide or risk of suicide a secret. If the young person doesn't want you to tell anyone about their suicidal thoughts, you should not agree, but give an explanation why, e.g. 'I care about you too much to keep a secret like this. You need help and I am here to help you get it.' Treat the person with respect and involve them in decisions about who else knows about the suicidal crisis.

If the person refuses to give permission to disclose information about their suicidal thoughts, then you may need to breach their confidentiality in order to ensure their safety. In doing so, you need to be honest and tell the person who you will be notifying.

Keep in mind that it is much better to have the person angry with you for sharing their suicidal thoughts without their permission, in order to obtain help, than to lose the person to suicide.

WHAT SHOULD I DO IF THE PERSON HAS ACTED ON SUICIDAL THOUGHTS?

If the suicidal person has already harmed themselves, administer first aid and call an ambulance.

Keep in mind that despite our best efforts, we may not be successful in preventing suicide. If the person dies, try not to blame yourself, and seek help if you need it.

TAKE CARE OF YOURSELF

After helping someone who is suicidal, make sure you take appropriate self-care. Providing support and assistance to a suicidal person is exhausting and it is therefore important to take care of yourself.

CONCLUSION

Suicide is often preventable, and simple helping strategies can enable young people to feel heard and supported. Arming yourself with suicide first aid skills can put you in a good position to help any young person in your life from acting on their thoughts of suicide and help them to get the mental health support they need.

Acknowledgements
The author would like to acknowledge Anna Ross, Anthony Jorm and Betty Kitchener, co-authors of the *Mental health first aid guidelines for suicidal thoughts and behaviours*.

Author biography

Dr Claire Kelly is the manager of youth programmes at Mental Health First Aid Australia. She has been a main contributor to the mental health first aid guidelines projects. Claire has experienced episodes of depression and anxiety since early adolescence, which has been a driver for her work.

www.mhfa.com.au

See also:

Chapter 1: Helping Young People Get Help for Mental Health Problems
Chapter 2: What to do in a Mental Health Crisis
Chapter 5: Depression in Young People
Chapter 6: Understanding Self-harm

Recommended websites:

Mental Health First Aid: www.mhfa.com.au or www.mhfaengland.org
NHS: www.nhs.uk/conditions/suicide
PAPYRUS (young suicide prevention): www.papyrus-uk.org
CALM (Campaign Against Living Miserably, for preventing male suicide): www.theclamzone.net

Further resources:

Childline:
    Helpline: 0800 1111

Samaritans:
    Helpline: 116 123

Further reading:

Australian Bureau of Statistics 2016, *3303.0 – Causes of Death Australia, 2015*, ABS, Canberra.

Hawton, K, van Heeringen, K 2009, 'Suicide', *The Lancet*, vol. 373, pp 1372–81.

Johnston, AK, Pirkis, JE & Burgess, PM 2009, 'Suicidal thoughts and behaviours among Australian adults: findings from the 2007 National Survey of Mental Health and Wellbeing', *Australian & New Zealand Journal of Psychiatry*, vol. 43, pp 635–43.

Lawrence D, Johnson S, Hakefost J, Boterhoven De Haan K, Sawyer M, Ainley J & Zubrick SR 2015, 'The Mental Health of Children and Adolescents', *Report on the Second Australian Child and Adolescent Survey of Mental Health and Wellbeing*, Department of Health, Canberra.

May, AM & Klonsky, ED 2013, 'Assessing motivations for suicide attempts: development and psychometric properties of the inventory of motivations for suicide attempts', *Suicide and Life-Threatening Behavior*, vol. 43, pp 532–46.

Mental Health First Aid Australia. *Suicidal Thoughts and Behaviours: First Aid Guidelines*, Mental Health First Aid Australia, Melbourne, 2014.

Ross, AM, Hart, LM, Jorm, AF, Kelly, CM & Kitchener, BA 2012, 'Development of key messages for adolescents on providing basic mental health first aid to peers: a Delphi consensus study', *Early intervention in psychiatry*, vol. 6, no. 3, pp 229–238.

Ross, AM, Kelly, CM & Jorm, AF 2014, 'Re-development of mental health first aid guidelines for suicidal ideation and behaviour: a Delphi study', *BMC Psychiatry*, vol. 14, p 241.

Rudd, MD, Berman, AL, Joiner, TE, Nock, MK, Silverman, MM, Mandrusiak, M, Van Orden, K & Witte, T 2006, 'Warning signs for suicide: theory, research, and clinical applications', *Suicide and Life-Threatening Behavior*, vol. 36, pp 255–262.

8. TOWARDS PREVENTION: UNDERSTANDING CHILD SEXUAL ASSAULT

Carol Ronken

Understanding the processes of grooming and offending behaviour helps us recognise the dynamics that impact on children and young people who have been affected by sexual assault. Moreover, in understanding these offending processes it becomes clearer how children and young people can be coerced into silence, or made to feel some responsibility for the offence. The better our understanding of this crime, the better we are equipped as parents, community members and people who work with children, to both protect and respond.

INTRODUCTION

Child sexual assault is a hidden but significant problem in every community in Australia. Experts estimate the prevalence ranging between one in five children to one in seven children experiencing some form of sexual assault before they reach the age of eighteen.[1] These include a continuum of offending behaviours; based on a review of research conducted on child sex assault cases over an eight-year period, researchers estimated that between 5 and 10 per cent of girls and up to 5 per cent of boys are exposed to penetrative sexual abuse, and up to three times this number are exposed to any type of sexual assault.[2]

The most vulnerable ages for children to be exposed to sexual assault appears to be between three and eight years of age[3] while the Australian Bureau of Statistics report that 25 per cent of victims of 'all' sexual assaults reported are aged between ten and fourteen. Less than one in ten of these children will tell.[4]

Research clearly shows that individuals who are sexually assaulted as children are far more likely to experience psychological problems often lasting into adulthood, including: Post Traumatic Stress Disorder, depression, substance abuse and relationship problems. Child sexual assault does not discriminate along lines of country, race, creed, socioeconomic status or gender; it crosses all boundaries to affect every community.

DEFINING CHILD SEXUAL ASSAULT

Traditionally, child sexual assault has been 'lumped in the same pot' as child abuse and neglect. However, while all forms of abuse and assault are harmful to children, it is important to take child sexual assault out of the 'pot' as the dynamics are fundamentally different. Recognising these differences and the varying ways necessary to respond to child sexual assault will enable this crime to be effectively addressed and prevented. Some of the important differences include:

- Acts of child abuse and neglect are generally unplanned, reactive, generally aligned with socioeconomic and/or family dysfunction issues and are comparatively predominant in areas of social disadvantage.
- Sexual assaults against children are almost always premeditated, involving predatory acts of grooming, manipulation, self-gratification and exploitation, and occur widely across the various socioeconomic areas.
- Child abuse and neglect more commonly involve the infliction of pain, violence and aggressive force.

- Child sexual assault more commonly involves manipulation, intimidation and inappropriate contact.
- Child abuse and neglect are perpetrated by a parent or primary caregiver in an estimated 90 per cent of cases.
- Child sexual assault is generally perpetrated by a male and is more likely to be perpetrated by someone known to the child or their family (research varies but commonly finds between 70 per cent and 90 per cent of the time[5]). Of those offenders known to the child, most commonly the offender is *not* living with the child.[6]
- Child abuse and neglect offences are almost always intra-familial.
- Child sex assault offences are commonly extra-familial as well as intra-familial.

Most countries have laws that prohibit sexual conduct with children and adolescents. Although these laws vary in details from state to state, they agree for the most part on what constitutes behaviour that is sexually exploitative.

DEFINITION

Broadly defined, child sexual assault includes:

Any act of inappropriately exposing or subjecting a child under the age of sixteen to sexual activity, contact or behaviour by an adult or by another child, for the purpose of gratification (sexual or otherwise) by the aggressor.

Often people think that child sexual assault refers only to rape. However, many survivors of child sexual assault may not experience penetrative offences such as rape. Instead they may experience a wide range of acts including genital exposure, fondling, forced touching, inappropriate kissing, oral sex or exposure to pornography.

Some examples of behaviours that constitute the sexual assault of children include:

- Elizabeth is ten. Her father comes into her room when she is sleeping and pulls her nightgown up so that he can rub her genital area with his hands.
- Tim is three. His mother keeps him in her bed and masturbates him until he has an erection.
- Steve and his friend Ben are invited to play with their neighbour's PlayStation. While playing, the neighbour suggests that the boys have a naked wrestling match while he takes pictures of them.
- Andrea is thinking about running away from home; her mother's boyfriend tries to kiss her while her mother is at work.
- Sally's teacher asks her to stay after class. While he is talking to her, he puts his arm around her and starts fondling her breast.
- Simon's football coach emails him pornographic stories involving men and young boys.
- Carl is fifteen. He babysits for his six-year-old niece. He gets into bed with her and makes her rub his penis.
- Tom's stepmother insists on giving him a bath, even though he is ten. She takes off her clothes and gets into the tub with him.

These are a few of the hundreds of examples of sexually exploitative behaviour. In each, we see a person who is taking advantage of someone younger and in a position of less power than they are.

As identified in these examples, offenders can be male or female; they may select a victim of the same sex or of the opposite sex; and they may be a family member, a friend or an acquaintance. Sometimes the offender may also be minor.

OFFENDERS AND GROOMING

Views that children are at risk predominantly from strangers have inhibited knowledge that most sexual assault of children occurs at the hands of someone the child knows, trusts and often loves.

We now know the people who most commonly sexually assault children are family members or individuals close to the family or child. Research shows that between 70 to 90 per cent of the time, the sexual assault involves an offender who is known and trusted by the child.[7] Strangers do indeed molest children. However, most of the time the offender is not the 'bogeyman' hiding in the bushes. It is instead a parent, a step-parent, a grandparent, an uncle, an aunt, a cousin, a neighbour, a family friend, a teacher, a member of the clergy, or someone else who is known to the child or their family.

Data from a sample of more than five hundred clients attending therapy at Australia's leading child protection organisation, Brave-hearts, over a five-year period indicated that approximately 97 per cent of offenders were known to the victim. Specifically, 40 per cent of offenders were a father or father figure living in the child's primary or secondary residence, 30 per cent were other family members and 27 per cent were known to the child and their family outside the home. Only 3 per cent were strangers. These figures are consistent with existing research showing the majority of offenders to be either related to or closely affiliated with the child.[8]

As previously mentioned, despite impressions gained from media reports of sexual crimes, child sexual assault is most often not violent. Usually it involves a process of grooming and contrived compliance based on trickery, manipulation and secrecy with a child to whom the offender often has a close relationship.[9] Understanding these offending components, it becomes clearer how easily children can become coerced into silence, or indeed made to feel some responsibility in the offence.

In order to effectively prevent the sexual assault of children, it is essential that offending behaviours and patterns are understood. Understanding the processes of grooming and offending helps in the recognition of the dynamics that impact on the children and young people.

There are many terminologies used to describe child sex offenders and offences, including:

- Child molesting/offenders: generally defines people who sexually offend against children or young people.
- Paedophiles: traditionally described as people who have a specific preference and/or attraction to prepubescent children (American Psychiatric Association). This is characterised by intense sexually arousing fantasies, urges, or behaviours involving sexual activity with a prepubescent child, typically aged thirteen or younger. You do not need to have committed an offence to be diagnosed as a paedophile.
- Incest: commonly refers to child sexual assault perpetrated by a family member.

Defining who is an offender and who is likely to sexually offend against a child is complex. There is no 'simple' or single profile of a child sex offender. Child sex offenders do not adhere to a particular stereotype. Offenders come from all walks of life, all family types and all ages.

The use of the terms *situational* and *preferential* offending offers a simple way to try to understand motivation for sexual offending (although this can be difficult to determine) and behaviour patterns.[10] It is important to be mindful that a preferential sex offender can have some of the motives and behaviour patterns of a situational sex offender and vice versa. The categories range from no true preference for children, and offending for a number of different reasons (e.g. power, aggression, social disorders), to a true sexual preference for children.

David Finkelhor, a US sociologist and Director of the Crimes Against Children Research Center, has developed what is termed the 'four preconditions of sex abuse',[11] which provides a model for understanding how the sexual assault of children occurs. The first precondition is the presence of an individual who has the motivation to sexually assault children. This motivation contains three components (any of which may be present but not all of which are required): emotional congruence, sexual arousal and blockage (an individual's inability to have a normal sexual relationship). Experience as a sexually assaulted child is a common feature leading to emotional congruence.

The second precondition is what Finkelhor terms internal inhibitors. Most individuals have internal inhibition of any intermittent desires to be sexually involved with children. When these internal inhibitors are absent, there is a greater likelihood of an abusive event. According to Finkelhor, alcohol and drugs are the two most common destroyers of internal inhibitors.

The third precondition for child sexual assault is the overcoming of external inhibitors. In families, the major external inhibitor is the presence of a protective parent. If the parent is not present or not protective then an individual with a motivation to sexually assault and no internal inhibitors finds the approach to a child easier.

The fourth precondition for child sexual assault is the breakdown of the child's resistance. Resistance may be taught either by parents or through education programmes and include the empowerment and build-up of resiliency and protective factors within the child and the child's environment. Overcoming external inhibitors and the resistance of a child are very much the intention of the grooming process.

Child sex offenders use a variety of tricks to 'groom' children or adolescents and, often, their primary caregivers. Common grooming techniques reported by offenders include:

- Building the child's trust: using presents, special attention, treats, spending time together and playing games with non-sexual physical contact.
- Favouritism: the offender treats the child as an adult; treating them differently and making them feel like a unique friend.
- Gaining the trust of the child's carer(s): careful to be seen as a close, caring and reliable relative or friend of the family.
- Isolation (from family, friends): to ensure secrecy and lessen chances of disclosure or belief.

- Intimidation and secrecy: the offender may use coercion, e.g. threatening looks and body language, glares, stalking and rules of secrecy.
- 'Testing the waters' or boundary violation: 'innocent' touching, gradually developing into 'accidental' sexual contact.
- Shaping the child's perceptions: the child is often confused as to what is acceptable and can take on self-blame for the situation, as his/her viewpoint can become totally distorted.[12]

It is widely acknowledged that people who sexually assault children engage in a cyclical pattern of behaviour. While there are variations among sex offenders in how they operate, the typical cycle involves starting with thoughts and feelings of the offender, moving to pro-offending thinking, then fantasy and rehearsal, targeting, grooming, offence, guilt and fear, maintaining secrecy and pretending to be normal. It is worth noting that this cycle would differ for situational (non-preferential) offenders, as well as for juvenile and female offenders.

THE SILENCE SURROUNDING CHILD SEXUAL ASSAULT

The perpetration of child sexual assault relies heavily on silencing the victim; in order to keep offending, perpetrators need secrecy. Offenders usually put a great deal of effort into ensuring that a child remains silent. Apart from promises, threats and bribes, offenders also take advantage of the child's powerlessness by presenting a distorted or false view of what is happening. Some of the ways offenders 'trick' children into secrecy include convincing the child that:

- They are somehow responsible.
- Others will blame them.
- They will be punished.
- They will be to blame if the offender goes to jail.
- They will be to blame if the family breaks up.
- They will be to blame if others in the family are upset.

- They are bad in some way and this is why the assault happened in the first place.
- They will not be 'special' anymore.
- No one would believe them if they told.

In childhood, the main factors influencing non-disclosure to family and friends are: when the offender is known to the child, when the offender is a family member, or when the child perceives there may be more negative outcomes (e.g. not being believed, family break-up), than positive outcomes (e.g. the abuse stops, safety).

One of the most commonly expressed reasons for not disclosing child sexual assault is a fear of not being believed.[13] Both children and adults report that this fear of non-belief is a major barrier to them disclosing to either trusted others or support services.[14]

It is so tough for anyone to disclose sexual assault. For children who do not have the language or the understanding of what has happened, it can be even more difficult, because:

- They often feel it is their fault because they let it happen.
- They feel guilty about their body's natural reaction to sexual activity (even though this is beyond their control).
- They feel disclosure may cause family problems or breakdowns.
- The offender may be someone they heavily rely on.
- They fear they will be blamed, punished or not believed.
- They fear they will be taken away from their homes and their families if they speak out.
- They fear disclosure will cause harm to someone or something they love and care for, such as family members or pets.

In fact, such is the pervasive nature of these fears and barriers to disclosure, even if a child has one or more supportive parents this does not necessarily increase their chances of disclosing their abuse history. In the case, as it so often is, where the abuse is from a parental figure, loved family member, or trusted family friend, the perceived likelihood of belief of the child is also severely compromised.[15]

SIGNS AND INDICATORS

While children often lack the cognitive capacity and the words to describe sexual assault, finding it exceptionally difficult to disclose, they may try to subtly open the conversation by saying, 'Do you like so and so? I don't', or 'I've got a secret'. Unfortunately, the more severe the degree of offending the less likely it is that the child/young person will disclose.[16] This is why it is important for all of us as protective adults to be vigilant for indicators of sexual assault.

There are a number of physical and behavioural symptoms that could be viewed as 'red flags' — a sign that something may be worrying the child. It should not be automatically assumed that harm is occurring; talking to the child may reveal something quite innocent. It is important, however, not to dismiss significant changes in behaviour, fears or physical symptoms.

Physical	Emotional/ Psychological	Behavioural	Social
Vaginal, penile or anal soreness, discharge or bleeding	Sexual knowledge outside expected for developmental age	Sexual behaviour outside that expected for age	Fear of being alone with a particular person
Psychosomatic symptoms	Personality changes	Regression in developmental milestones	Withdrawal from friends
Vague symptoms of illness such as headache or tummy ache	Recurrent nightmares	Increased conduct problems	Changes to the child's social network
Bruises, bite marks or other injuries to breasts, buttocks, lower abdomen	Increased psychological symptoms	Fearful, anxious, regressed or avoidant behaviour with certain stimuli	Deterioration in academic functioning
Development of eating disorders	Self-harming	Risk-taking behaviours	Overattention to adults of a particular sex

IMPACT AND EFFECTS

Children and adolescents who have been sexually assaulted can suffer a range of psychological and behavioural problems, from mild to severe, in both the short and long term.

The initial or short-term effects of sexual assault usually occur during and within two years of the termination of the assault.[17] These effects vary depending upon the circumstances of the offending, the child's developmental stage, whether or not they have disclosed and the response to any attempts to disclose.[18] Typical presentations at Bravehearts may include regressive behaviours, sleep disturbances, eating problems, behavioural and/ or performance problems at school and non-participation in school and social activities.

The negative effects of child sexual assault can affect the survivor for many years and into adulthood, including depression and self-destructive behaviours.[19] Many survivors also encounter problems in their adult relationships and in their adult sexual functioning.

Re-victimisation is also a common phenomenon among people harmed as children. Research has shown that child sexual assault survivors are more likely to be the victims of rape or to be involved in physically abusive relationships as adults.[20]

Despite all this, it is really important to understand that the impacts and effects of child sexual assault can be reduced. Many survivors are able to live perfectly happy and secure lives. Children and adults who are supported and believed when they speak out are less likely to endure long-term negative impacts.[21] The response of others to disclosed or suspected harm is a crucial factor.

Some of the common effects of child sexual assault seen in children and young people include:

- psychosomatic responses
- psychiatric disorders
- long-lasting emotional problems
- youth suicide
- regression
- sleeping and eating disorders
- lack of self-esteem
- nightmares

- self-harming/mutilation
- self-hatred
- promiscuous behaviour
- aggression
- behavioural changes.

A wide variety of effects that can be seen in the long term include:

- the development of violent behaviour
- the development of criminal behaviour
- long-term psychiatric problems
- suicide
- post-traumatic stress
- sexual difficulties
- inability to form lasting relationships
- a serious lack of self-confidence
- marital problems
- poor parenting skills
- alcohol and substance misuse.

MYTHS, FACTS AND STATISTICS

Myths are often used to explain the unexplainable, to make sense out of things that make no sense. Sometimes people use myths to protect themselves from painful realities.

There are a number of myths and fallacies that surround the issue of child sexual assault, because the reality of the problem is incomprehensible and frightening to many. These myths affect appropriate responses not only from individuals and the general community, but also can influence responses from the child protection and justice systems, as well as counselling and support services. Examples of some of the common myths and misinformation that pervade this issue are discussed below.

MYTH #1: Sex offenders are strangers and dirty old men.

REALITY: Children are often warned not to talk to strangers in the hope that this will protect them from child sexual assault. Statistics suggest that around 90 per cent of sexual assault is perpetrated by someone known to the child and/or their family.[22] Rather than attacking from the bushes, the sexual offender uses his position and relationship with a child to control and manipulate.

Sex offenders are both male and female, all ages and from all walks of life, although statistics show that the average age of sex offenders is thirty-six years of age.[23]

MYTH #2: People who sexually assault their own children are not a danger to other children.

REALITY: For many child sex offenders, child sexual assault is rarely a single offence, and a person who offends against their own children may offend against other children.

MYTH #3: Child sexual assault is rare.

REALITY: One in three girls and one in six boys will be sexually victimised by the age of eighteen.[24] No one knows the exact number of victims of childhood sexual assault. Because the injuries in sexual assault are primarily emotional rather than physical, it is less likely that someone other than the victim will be aware of the assaults. Unless the victim tells someone, the sexual assault will not be reported and the victim may continue to be victimised.

MYTH #4: Child sexual assault is not harmful to children.

REALITY: Studies show that sexual assault has many harmful effects on children. Survivors often need help and support to overcome these effects. Sexual assault of children often causes long-lasting emotional problems. Young victims often experience sleep problems, nightmares, nervous reactions, learning difficulties, depression, loss of self-esteem, behavioural difficulties, problems with peers, and the list goes on. A lot of children are frightened, especially when they have been threatened; many are confused, because they might enjoy some aspects of the relationship and may feel guilty about it, or they are too scared to tell anyone.

Not all victims experience all of these effects. The occurrence and intensity of the effects of sexual assault seem, from the research, to be directly related to the closeness of the relationship between the victim and the perpetrator, the age of the victims when sexual contact began and the duration of the abuse.[25]

MYTH #5: It's really the parents' fault, because they should protect the child.
REALITY: Parents are often accused of 'not protecting the child' in cases of sexual assault, whether or not they know about it. This attitude shifts the blame and allows the real offenders to avoid responsibility for their actions.

MYTH #6: A reason some people use to excuse child sexual offenders is to argue that the offender was abused as a child and therefore it's not their fault because they can't help it.
REALITY: As discussed early in the section on offenders, Finkelhor's preconditions for sexual offending recognises that the motivation to offend may result from being sexually assaulted as a child. In addition, the absence of internal inhibitions to sexually offend against a child may be related to childhood experiences. However, research has shown that most people who have been sexually assaulted do not go on to sexually assault their own or other people's children.[26]

MYTH #7: Men who sexually assault boys are homosexual.
REALITY: Most men who molest boys are heterosexual.[27] There is no evidence that homosexual men sexually assault boys any more than heterosexual men.

MYTH #8: Incest and sexual assault only occurs in poor families.

REALITY: Incest and sexual assault may occur in families rich or poor, large or small, well educated or not.

MYTH #9: The child never said no, or tried to stop the sexual assault, so it's the child's fault if they're assaulted.

REALITY: For many reasons children may not be able to say 'no'. The common anxiety response to freeze may prevent a child from saying no. It is always the offenders who are responsible, as children do not have the ability to consent.

MYTH #10: Children and young people lie or fantasise about sexual assault.

REALITY: Some adults prefer to believe this. Research has shown that in 98 per cent of reports by children, their statements were found to be true.[28]

It is extremely unlikely that minors will lie about sexual assault. The reality is that it takes a great deal of courage for victims of child sexual assault to come forward. When they do share their secret with someone, they should be believed. If the sexual assault did not occur, discrepancies in the repeated story will begin to surface. The made-up disclosure, though rare, cannot be ignored. It is an indication of some issue in the child or young person's life. Counselling is an absolute necessity in such cases.

MYTH #11: If a child discloses sexual assault and then retracts their statement, they must be lying.

REALITY: Enormous pressure is mounted on a child following a disclosure. Consequences of a disclosure can include family breakdown, distressed parents and a lack of support. A child may believe that if they say they were lying, then things will return to normal. However, an offender will not stop offending, and may become more aggressive knowing that if a child discloses again, they will not be believed.

MYTH #12: It's not the sexual assault that is harmful, it's all the fuss that the adults, child protection authorities and legal systems make that is the problem.

REALITY: In some cases intervention by legal, medical and welfare personnel can be distressing; however, this shouldn't be used as an excuse by people to not speak out and to allow sexual assault to continue. In surveys of survivors, most children describe negative effects during the time they were sexually assaulted.

The original version of this chapter was published in McKillop, N., Ronken, C., & Vidler S., *The Bravehearts Toolbox for Practitioners Working with Child Sexual Assault.* Bowen Hills [Qld]: Australian Academic Press, 2014.

Author biography

Carol Ronken worked as a researcher and Associate Lecturer at Griffith University in the School of Criminology and Criminal Justice before joining Bravehearts in early 2003. With a BA (Psych) and Masters Applied Sociology (Social Research), Carol is the Head of Research and Policy Development for Bravehearts. In 2011 she received an award from the Queensland Police Service Child Protection and Investigation Unit for her contribution to child protection. Carol has co-authored *The Bravehearts Toolbox for Practitioners Working with Child Sexual Assault* (Australian Academic Press, 2011).

www.bravehearts.org.au

See also:
Chapter 4: Anxiety in Young People
Chapter 5: Depression in Young People

 For more online resources visit:
generationnext.com.au/handbook

ALCOHOL AND DRUGS

Talking About Alcohol and Drugs   133

Supporting a Young Person in their Decision
Not to Use Alcohol or Other Drugs   150

Teens, Parties and Alcohol: A Practical Guide
to Keeping Them Safe   166

9. TALKING ABOUT ALCOHOL AND DRUGS

Siobhan Lawler, Nicola Newton, Katrina Champion & Lexine Stapinski

To prevent the short- and long-term harm that can be associated with early initiation to alcohol and other drug use, it is important to communicate with young people so they know the facts about these substances and how to stay safe. Equipping young people with up-to-date, evidence-based information and support empowers them to make informed decisions about drug and alcohol use.

INTRODUCTION – WHAT SCHOOL STAFF AND PARENTS NEED TO KNOW ABOUT ALCOHOL AND OTHER DRUGS

A drug is a substance that affects the way the body functions when it is used. Common drugs include alcohol, tobacco, and over-the-counter and prescription medications. Some drugs, such as methamphetamine and heroin, are forbidden by law. Drugs affect people differently as their effects are influenced by many factors, making them unpredictable. In the case of illegal drugs, the effects are difficult to predict as the potency and/or combination of substances used can vary greatly. This unpredictability makes them especially risky for young people.

FACTORS THAT INFLUENCE THE EFFECTS OF A DRUG

- The type and purity of the drug.
- How much is consumed.
- Where the person is when the drug is being used.
- What the person is doing while using the drug.
- Individual characteristics such as body size and health vulnerabilities.
- How many different drugs are taken at one time.

GLOSSARY OF IMPORTANT TERMS

Depressants are drugs that slow down the central nervous system and the messages that go between the brain and the body. These drugs decrease people's concentration and slow down their ability to respond. The name 'depressant' suggests that these drugs can make a person feel depressed, but this is not always the case. The term depressant purely refers to the effect of slowing down the central nervous system. Some examples of depressants include: alcohol, opioids (e.g. heroin), barbiturates and GHB.

Stimulants (also referred to as psychostimulants) are drugs that stimulate the central nervous system and speed up the messages going between the brain and the body. These drugs typically increase energy, heart rate and appetite. Some examples of psychostimulants include: methamphetamine (speed, ice, base), cocaine, dexamphetamine, caffeine, nicotine, ecstasy (MDMA).

Hallucinogens are drugs which typically alter how a person perceives the world, including how they see, hear, taste, feel or smell. Hallucinogens can also cause people to see, hear, smell, taste and feel things that are not there at all. Some examples of hallucinogens include: ketamine, magic mushrooms, LSD, acid.

Polydrug use is when a person mixes different drugs together, or takes more than one different kind of drug at the same time. Combining drugs in this way carries extra risks and can be very dangerous. The more drugs a person takes (or is affected by) at a time, the more chance there is of something going wrong. An example of polydrug use would be smoking cannabis while drinking alcohol or mixing alcohol with energy drinks. The effect of polydrug use depends on which drugs are mixed together, and is influenced by the types of drugs used, the individual person who is using the drug and the setting where it is taken. Combining drugs that have the same physical effects (e.g. two or more stimulants, or two or more depressants) is especially dangerous because it increases the impact on the normal functioning of the brain and body.

The **'comedown' or 'crash'** phase is the period when the drug effects start to wear off. Just like getting a hangover from drinking alcohol, taking illegal drugs can have negative after-effects which vary depending on the type of drug(s) used. They might include feelings of depression, insomnia, extreme tiredness, irritability and anxiety, to name just a few. The comedown phase can last anywhere from a few hours to a day or so after initially taking the drug. This is different to withdrawal effects (a sign that a person is addicted).

Dependence or addiction to drugs can happen when people use drugs regularly, and so become physically and/or psychologically dependent on using the drug. They can develop tolerance, which means that after using a drug over time, they need to take more of the drug to get the same effect.

Withdrawal effects happen to some people when they stop using a drug that they have become dependent on. Withdrawal effects can last for days to many weeks, depending on the type of drug and how dependent the person is on that drug. Withdrawal effects (or symptoms) may include feelings of anxiety, depression, restlessness, irritability and aggression. On top of this, withdrawal can also cause muscle spasms, headaches, muscle cramps, diarrhoea, vomiting and cravings for the drug.

HOW COMMON IS DRUG USE AMONG YOUNG PEOPLE?

It may be shown differently by the media, but the truth is that the majority of young people have never tried an illegal drug. This is an important message to communicate, because young people may be more inclined to experiment if they think most of their friends use drugs.

The drugs most commonly used by young people between the ages of fourteen and nineteen are alcohol (54 per cent) and tobacco (16.2 per cent). Cannabis is the most commonly used illegal drug (15 per cent). Other illegal drugs, such as ecstasy (MDMA, 3 per cent), synthetic cannabis (2.7 per cent), hallucinogens (2.4 per cent), methamphetamine (2 per cent), opiates (1 per cent) and cocaine (1 per cent) are much less common among this age group.

Although the majority of young people do not use drugs, for those who do, the impact can be significant. Research suggests that the earlier a young person starts to use alcohol and/or other drugs, the greater the risk of short- and long-term problems, including injury and accidents, poor school performance, and risk of developing mental health problems such as anxiety or depression. Teenage substance use can also lead to substance use disorders. On average, 12.5 per cent of young people between the ages of sixteen and twenty-four will experience a substance use disorder, with higher rates among young men (16 per cent) than young women (10 per cent).

CAN THESE PROBLEMS BE PREVENTED?

The teenage years are an important period, and mark the typical age that a young person first encounters alcohol and/or other drugs. Peer and social factors also become highly influential at this time. To prevent the short- and long-term harms that can be associated with alcohol and other drug use, it is important to communicate effectively with young people so they know the facts about these substances and how to stay safe. Equipping young people with up-to-date, non-sensationalist, evidence-based information and support empowers them to make informed decisions about alcohol and other drug use.

The good news is that as parents, teachers and school staff, there are effective strategies you can implement to help protect young people from harm relating to drug use. A number of drug education curriculum programs have been developed and tested in the school setting, with positive results including reduced student use of alcohol and other drugs. Parents can also help to prevent harm relating to alcohol and other drugs by being a good role model, establishing clear expectations and good communication. Even small changes can have a significant impact. For example, research suggests that the risk of a substance use disorder can be reduced by 10 per cent for each year that use is delayed in adolescence. This is a seemingly small effect in the short term that has a very big impact in the longer term.

COMMON MYTHS ABOUT ALCOHOL AND OTHER DRUGS

There are a lot of misconceptions about alcohol and other drugs. This is one reason why it is important to discuss alcohol and other drug use with young people – to ensure they are equipped with the facts, rather than misinformation conveyed by peers or the media. You may find it useful to discuss some of the myths about alcohol and drugs, and do some 'myth busting'.

COMMON MYTHS AND MISCONCEPTIONS

These have been tested against research-based facts and statistics.

Myth: Everybody is doing it.
Fact: It may be shown differently by the media, but the truth is that the majority of young people have never tried an illegal drug.

Myth: Alcohol makes it easier for people to socialise.

Fact: Alcohol in small quantities can make people feel more relaxed and sociable. However, alcohol is a 'downer'. Drinking too much alcohol can make people want to withdraw from others, or feel aggressive – which doesn't help much with improving social relationships. Drinking too much can also lead to feeling sick or vomiting, resulting in some very socially embarrassing moments!

To find out more, read our **Alcohol: Factsheet***.

Myth: It is safe to drive after using cannabis.

Fact: Using cannabis can increase the likelihood of a car crash by 300 per cent. Cannabis slows down thinking and reflexes, and reduces concentration and coordination. As a result, cannabis affects performance on a range of tasks and activities.

To find out more, read our **Cannabis: Factsheet***.

Myth: Methamphetamine is made in a controlled lab environment.

Fact: Because it is illegal, methamphetamine is commonly manufactured in unregulated laboratories that mix various forms of amphetamines and other chemicals to cut costs and boost potency.

See our **Methamphetamine: Factsheet*** for more information.

Myth: 'Legal Highs' are safe as they are legal.

Fact: Simply because something is sold in a shop or online, or as a legal/alternative 'high', it does not mean that it is harmless or safe to use. Taking these drugs is like a roll of the dice – they haven't been around long enough to know what the immediate risks are or what might happen later in life to people who use them. **Many drugs sold as 'legal highs' (also called 'party pills', 'research chemicals' or 'plant food') are actually illegal, or will soon be made illegal, because of their health risks.**

To find out more, read our **'Legal Highs': Factsheet***.

Myth: Teenagers are too young to get addicted.

Fact: Dependence (addiction) can happen at any age. Even unborn children can become dependent because of their mothers' drug use.

Myth: The logo on a pill is a good indicator of its ingredients and how strong it will be.

Fact: A logo or stamp is no guarantee of a pill's quality or purity: two pills that look the same may have very different effects as they can come from different sources and have different ingredients. You can never be sure what chemicals are in a pill or how you will be affected.

To find out more, read our **Ecstasy and Pills: Factsheet***.

*These factsheets are available on the Positive Choices portal: **www.positivechoices.org.au/resources/factsheets**

WHAT CAN PARENTS DO TO PREVENT DRUG-RELATED HARMS?

As a parent or guardian, you have a big impact on a teenager's life and the decisions they make. Research has shown there are many ways in which parents can minimise the chances that an adolescent will use illegal drugs, or experience harm from their use.

1. Be a good role model

Your behaviour and attitude towards alcohol, cigarettes and drugs have a big influence on your child's behaviour, so it is important to set a good example. Parental disapproval of early alcohol use is associated with reduced adolescent alcohol use and positive attitudes towards alcohol can increase risk for young people. It's important that you talk about alcohol and other drug use with your children, but it's also important to be cautious and conscious of the messages you might be sending. How you talk about alcohol to your children matters; even when the intention is to caution, warn or educate teenagers about the harms through storytelling and scare tactics, this can unintentionally normalise the issue and if you go too far, they won't believe what you are saying. Avoid contradictions between what you tell them and what you do, and try to demonstrate ways to have fun and deal with problems that don't involve drugs or alcohol.

2. Be involved in their lives

Be sure to regularly spend time with your child where you can give them your undivided attention; you could set up a routine of having meals together or helping them with their homework. Get involved and show an interest in their hobbies and activities. Have internet access in a central area in the house. If they go out, ask them about where they are going and who they are going with and make this discussion a regular part of your conversation. Simply knowing who your child is with and where they are can help reduce risk.

Your children's friends influence their behaviour, so it is natural to want to help your child choose the right friends and to get to know them. Invite them to your house, or talk to them if you pick your child up from school or after-school activities. Get to know their parents as well, as they can provide a support network to look out for the safety of your children. If you have good reason to believe your child's friends are involved in drugs, be prepared to support your child to find a new set of friends by engaging them in some new activities.

3. Establish and maintain good communication

Let your child know that you are always ready and willing to talk and listen. Ask open-ended questions and encourage them to share their thoughts, feelings and opinions to show you value what they think. This will encourage them to be honest and not just say what they think you want to hear. When talking to them, try not to lecture them; it is important to listen to their thoughts and concerns and offer help and support. Try to make yourself available most of the time. For example, make sure your child can contact you easily if they are at a party.

What to look out for?

Some signs and behaviours that may be associated with drug use include: withdrawal from family and friends; a change in friends; a drop in grades at school; signs of depression; hostility; an increase in borrowing money; evidence of drug paraphernalia or missing prescription drugs.

However, many of these behavioural changes are common as part of normal development through adolescence, so it is important not to assume they are related to drug use. If you suspect your child may be affected by drug use, arrange a time to talk with them when you will have some privacy and won't be interrupted. Prepare by gathering factual information so that you are informed about drug effects and risks, and ready to articulate your concerns calmly in a supportive, non-confrontational manner.

WHAT CAN SCHOOL STAFF DO TO PREVENT DRUG-RELATED HARMS?

Most people will first encounter alcohol and/or other drugs during the teenage years, either at school, at home or through TV or other media channels. School staff and others working closely with young people can have a significant influence on the extent to which students feel they belong or are part of a school community. The conversations you have with young people about drug use can be important opportunities for education, prevention and early intervention. It is understandable to be hesitant about how to approach these conversations, or unsure of the facts relating to alcohol and other drug use. You can inform yourself about different drug types, their effects and risks by accessing the comprehensive information available from Talk to Frank: www.talktofrank.com. Being prepared with accurate, non-sensationalist and factual information will help you communicate with young people in an effective and non-confrontational manner.

Each school has its own policy around alcohol and other drug-related matters, and when suspecting drug use duty-of-care procedures must be followed. If a student is experiencing problems related to drug use, a staff member or school counsellor who is trained in dealing with these issues may be able to assist in providing the necessary resources or referrals. The good news is that effective approaches to prevention, early intervention and treatment of alcohol and other drug use are available.

How to foster a positive relationship between students and their school

Research suggests that young people who have a strong sense of belonging and feel they are part of a school community are less likely to become involved in high-risk health behaviours such as early substance use. School staff and other professionals working with young people can help to encourage a positive attitude towards school in the following ways:

- Setting clear rules and boundaries that are consistently enforced in a reasonable and measured manner.
- Keeping an open mind and asking students for their opinions.
- Giving praise and reward for students' good behaviour, achievements and accomplishments.
- Encouraging a constructive use of time.
- Modelling a sense of optimism and a positive view of learning.
- Encouraging participation in extracurricular activities.
- Encouraging reading for pleasure outside of school hours.
- Being a good listener.

HOW TO TALK TO A YOUNG PERSON ABOUT ILLEGAL DRUGS

Parents and school staff are the primary sources of contact for young people seeking advice or help for drug use issues. The conversations that you have with young people about drug use can be important opportunities to educate them, prevent future problems, and/ or assist them in accessing support. It is understandable to feel concerned about how to approach these conversations, and school staff or health professionals trained in dealing with drug problems (e.g. counsellor, psychologist or nurse) may be able to provide advice or assist in obtaining necessary resources or medical referrals. School staff should also familiarise themselves with any relevant duty-of-care procedures. Following are some tips to help you communicate effectively with young people about drug use.

Stick to the facts

Studies show that young people's attitudes are shaped by the way adults speak about alcohol and other drug use. Exaggerating or sensationalising language can be counterproductive when teenagers perceive they are not being given an accurate picture. Likewise, recounting personal stories can have the effect of normalising or enhancing positive views of alcohol and drug use, even when the intention is to caution young people. Behavioural changes are a good starting point for discussion, for example, 'I noticed you haven't been yourself lately...' Before approaching these conversations, do some research to ensure you are equipped with accurate information, and have a clear message in mind that conveys the risks and the facts about drug use.

Correct common misperceptions

Only three in one hundred young persons aged fourteen to nineteen tried ecstasy last year.

Research suggests that social influences such as friends and family are powerful predictors of alcohol and other drug use in adolescence. Young people often overestimate the rates of alcohol and other drug use among their friends and assume that 'everyone is doing it'. A simple but effective way to correct this misperception is to provide accurate facts about drug use in Australia. For example, the national surveys of drug use tell us that most teenagers (ninety-six out of one hundred) have never tried ecstasy (MDMA). Providing young people with information in this way helps to reinforce the message that most young people do not use drugs.

Emphasise rewarding alternatives

Emphasise that there are other things to do that are rewarding and fun. Encourage young people to make the most out of the extracurricular activities (i.e. creative activities, team sport) offered within and outside the school community. Drawing attention to a young person's strengths and providing support to become involved in related activities can increase a student's self-esteem and foster a positive relationship with school – which studies suggest can reduce the potential for drug abuse.

Don't be judgemental

When a young person is going through a challenging time, they are likely to shut down if they suspect you are patronising or not listening to them. Make it clear that you are trying to understand their concerns, but also be ready for negative reactions. Ask questions rather than making assumptions about a student's drug use. Be sure to listen and express your concerns in a supportive, non-confrontational manner. Avoid putting the blame on them by saying things like 'you're stressing me out with your drug use' and instead use statements including 'I', for example, 'I feel concerned about your drug use'. Be prepared for a negative reaction. One reason for this may be that they do not view their drug use as a problem. Be sure to stay calm and reasonable. Don't let it turn into an argument. Be trustworthy and supportive so they know that they can rely on you in a time of need. Remind them that we are all human and that we all have problems so that they are not too hard on themselves. Let them know that help is available.

Seeking professional help may be the next step. You can consult the school counsellor, who will be able to support you in your efforts to communicate with a student. See the end of this chapter for a list of places available to help people of all ages with any drug issues.

WHY DO YOUNG PEOPLE USE DRUGS?

An insight into the pressures young people face and possible reasons for drug use can help you to respond in a constructive way. Below are some of the reasons young people give for using drugs, and some ideas for starting conversations with them.

'Someone had some and I just thought I'd try it'	• Ask if they knew what they were taking and discuss the effects of the drug. • Try to find out if they felt pressured, and if so, talk about ways to handle similar situations in the future.
'I always wanted to try that stuff'	• Ask what made that particular drug appealing, and what they expected to get from it. • Ask whether it was what they expected, and discuss some of the risks that might be involved.
'All my friends were doing it so I thought why not?'	• Ask if they felt safe because their friends were using it. • Ask why they thought their friends used the drug. • Explore the importance of being able to make their own choices, even if these choices are different from those of their friends.
'It made me feel really good'	• Find out how they have been feeling in general, as this may be a good time to offer help and to find out if there is anything else going on, or if they want to talk about another issue. • Talk about less risky and healthier ways of feeling good.
'All my problems from school, at home and in life just went away'	• Let them know that you'd like to talk about any problems and work together to find a way to make things better. • Discuss whether the problems returned after the effects of the drug wore off, highlight that using drugs only makes the problems disappear for a while.
'It gave me more confidence'	• Let them know there are other, less risky, ways to gain confidence. • Share similar experiences where you found it difficult in social situations and explain things you did to gain more confidence. • Consider ways in which you can help improve their confidence and self-esteem.
'I don't want to talk about it'	• If they don't want to discuss their use with you, offer to help them find someone else to talk to. • Reassure them that what you want is what is best for them and understand if they would prefer to speak to someone else outside of the situation.

HELPING SOMEONE WHO HAS TAKEN AN ILLEGAL DRUG

The majority of people never use drugs, but it is important for people to know how to assist someone if a drug-related emergency happens.

Drugs are unpredictable; they can affect people in different ways and as there is no quality control for illegal drugs there is no way of knowing their content or strength.

CALL 999 OR 112 FOR AN AMBULANCE IMMEDIATELY IF THERE IS EVEN THE SLIGHTEST RISK THAT SOMEONE IS HAVING AN UNUSUAL REACTION TO A DRUG

A parent or guardian will only be notified if the person is under the age of eighteen and taken to hospital. Police will only be notified if there is a risk to the young person's personal safety or if someone dies. It is important that young people aren't afraid to reach out for help.

Below is a guide to assisting a person in the following situations.

Panic attacks: These can happen due to the increased feelings of paranoia, anxiety and hallucinations that illegal drugs can bring on. These can be very frightening at the time, but it is important to know that these usually pass with time.

What are some of the signs?
- Sweating and shaking.
- Chest pains and difficulty breathing.
- Increased heart rate.
- Sense of impending death.
- Dizziness, headaches and light-headedness.
- 'Spaced-out' and non-responsive.

What to do if someone has a panic attack:
- Calm them down and reassure them that the feeling will pass.
- Take them somewhere cool and quiet away from crowds and bright lights.
- Encourage them to relax and take long, slow, deep breaths.
- If they pass out due to over-breathing, lay them down, raise their legs above their head by propping their ankles on your

shoulders. Ensure they have plenty of fresh air, and they should recover after a couple of minutes.

Overheating and dehydration: There is a serious risk of overheating and dehydration when people dance for hours and do not maintain their fluids. Stimulants such as ecstasy and methamphetamine will increase the body temperature, and this problem can be made worse if taken with alcohol as it will further dehydrate the body. Those who take stimulants should try to drink half a litre of water every hour, but make sure not to drink too much too quickly.

What are some of the signs?
- Feeling hot, unwell, lethargic, faint or dizzy.
- Inability to talk properly.
- Headache.
- Vomiting.
- Inability to urinate or urine becoming thick and dark.
- Not sweating even when dancing.
- Fainting, collapsing or convulsing.

What to do if someone becomes overheated and dehydrated:
- Take them somewhere cool and quiet such as the first-aid area or 'chill-out' room.
- Get the person some cold water and get them to sip it slowly.
- Make sure someone stays with them.
- Give them salted foods like crisps or peanuts to replace salts lost through sweating.
- Fan them to cool them down.
- If symptoms persist or get worse, seek first aid immediately, call 000, or take them to the nearest emergency department.

Feeling very drowsy: If someone becomes very drowsy from using drugs they could fall asleep and lose consciousness. It is important to keep them awake while waiting for the ambulance.

What to do if someone becomes very drowsy:

- Call an ambulance, but make sure they are not left on their own.
- Keep them awake; make them walk around or make them talk to you.
- Don't give them coffee or try to shock them.
- If they aren't responsive or lose consciousness, put them in the recovery position.

Fits or seizures (convulsions): large amounts of alcohol and some drugs can cause convulsions, otherwise known as a fit or seizure.

What to do if someone starts convulsing:

- Call an ambulance.
- Clear the area of any nearby harmful objects.
- Loosen any tight clothing.
- Cushion their head.
- It is important not to put anything in their mouth or to try to restrict their movement.
- Once the fit has finished, check their breathing and put them in the recovery position.

Acknowledgements

The authors would like to acknowledge the contribution of Professor Maree Teesson to the development of this chapter. Some information and images in this chapter have been adapted from the Climate Schools programme (www.climateschools.com.au) and the Positive Choices national portal (www.positivechoices.org.au). Positive Choices is funded by the Australian Government Department of Health.

Authors' biographies

Siobhan, Nicola, Katrina and Lexine are all affiliated with the NHMRC Centre of Research Excellence in Mental Health and Substance Use at the National Drug and Alcohol Research Centre, UNSW in Sydney.

Siobhan Lawler has been Research Assistant and Social Media Manager for the Positive Choices initiative since 2015. It provides evidence-based drug education and prevention resources and training for school communities. Associate Professor Nicola Newton is Director of Prevention. She leads a program of research developing and evaluating innovative approaches to the prevention of substance use, mental health problems and risky health behaviours in adolescents. Dr Katrina Champion is an NHMRC Early Career Fellow. She has been closely involved in the development, evaluation and translation of the Climate Schools substance use prevention programmes. Dr Lexine Stapinski is a Senior Research Fellow and Clinical Psychologist. She leads the Positive Choices project, a national initiative to improve dissemination of evidence-based drug prevention across Australia.

www.ndarc.med.unsw.edu.au

See also:

Chapter 10: Supporting a Young Person in their Decision Not to Use Alcohol or Other Drugs

Chapter 11: Teens, Parties and Alcohol: A Practical Guide to Keeping Them Safe

Further resources:

Talk to Frank: www.talktofrank.com

National Drug Prevention Alliance: www.drugprevent.org.uk

Drinkaware: www.drinkaware.co.uk

NHS: www.nhs.uk/Livewell/alcohol

NHS: www.nhs.uk/Livewell/drugs

Alcohol Concern: www.alcoholconcern.org.uk

HIT: www.hit.org.uk

Mind: www.mind.org.uk

Further reading:

Newton, N, Rodriguez, D, Teesson, M, Black, E, Rainsford, C, Allsop, S, McBride, N, Swift, W, Bryant, Z, Kay-Lambkin, F, Chapman, C, Reda, B, Stapinski, L & Slade, T, 2014, *Illegal drugs: What you need to know (Student version)*, NDARC, Sydney.

Newton, N, Rodriguez, et al 2014, *Illegal drugs: What you need to know (Parent version)*, NDARC, Sydney.

Newton, N et al 2014. *Illegal drugs: What you need to know (Teacher version)*, NDARC, Sydney.

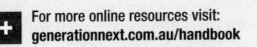

For more online resources visit:
generationnext.com.au/handbook

10. SUPPORTING A YOUNG PERSON IN THEIR DECISION NOT TO USE ALCOHOL OR OTHER DRUGS

Paul Dillon

Most people are aware that illicit drug use is not the norm among our teens, but it is also important to acknowledge that growing numbers of young Australians are choosing not to drink alcohol. This chapter examines why young people make such a choice, and will suggest how those around them can best support their decision, with an emphasis on alcohol and being a 'non-drinker'.

INTRODUCTION

We live in a world that thrives on focusing on the negative, particularly when it comes to our young people. If you believe everything you see, read and hear in the media, it would be difficult not to think that the current generation of teens is one of the worst in history, with rarely a day going past without headlines such as 'young people on the rampage', 'teen crime spree' or 'youth crime rate soars'. When it comes to alcohol and using other drugs, many adults believe that the situation is so much worse than when they were young. Certainly, there are many young people who drink and a minority who choose to experiment with illegal drugs, with some having significant issues that should not be ignored – but what about all those teens who make the decision not to take part in these activities?

The greatest problem with focusing only on those who do drink alcohol or use other drugs is that the more we do it, the more that group is perceived as the 'norm', i.e. that is what 'everyone' does. Of course, it is important to be realistic and acknowledge the problems that do exist, but they need to be presented in a context and, unfortunately, that is rarely, if ever, done. An example of how easily a context can be provided is as follows, in relation to methamphetamine use in Australia.

'Ice' use among methamphetamine users has indeed doubled in recent years but it is important to remember that 93 per cent of Australians have never used the drug.

When we don't talk about the majority and, in doing so, provide a context, it affects how the community perceives the issue. Due to the great focus on those young people who drink alcohol – particularly those who drink to excess – many adults, especially parents, believe that all teenagers drink and that it is simply inevitable that their child will go through this 'rite of passage' and there is nothing they can do to prevent it. More importantly, however, those young people who choose not to drink start to question their choices and begin to worry that something is wrong with them: 'Everybody else is doing it, why aren't I?'

Most adults are aware that illicit drug use is not the norm among school-based young people in Australia. Rates of recent illicit drug use are lower than in the late 1990s and although there is an increasing range of drugs available, there is no evidence to suggest that use is on the rise. Due to the illicit nature of these drugs and their perceived harm, the vast majority of adults send fairly strong messages to young people about their concerns and support them in their decision not to use these substances. Unfortunately, the same cannot always be said about alcohol.

Alcohol. It plays a major role in many people's lives when it comes to socialising and is not only regarded as 'socially acceptable' but 'socially expected', i.e. if you don't drink, there must be something wrong with you. We drink alcohol to celebrate, to commiserate, to relax, to have fun. In fact, alcohol is central to almost any social gathering or event. Although there are few, if any, parents who want their child to start drinking alcohol, particularly in their early teens, many believe that it is indeed a 'rite of passage' and there is little they can do to prevent it. There are also those who become concerned when their teen doesn't drink as they believe 'he/she won't fit in' and as a result will find themselves socially excluded.

It is interesting, therefore, that even within a culture where drinking has become socially expected, we have a growing number of adolescents choosing not to drink alcohol. Not just reducing the amount they drink (and the numbers drinking less are increasing as well), but not drinking at all. There is a range of reasons that have been suggested for this and this chapter will discuss some of those, but whatever the motivation, this group of non-drinkers need the support of the adults around them if they choose this path. Although there are particular cultural groups where illicit drug use is more likely to occur (e.g. nightclub dance culture and ecstasy use), it is not the social norm across the general population. Alcohol use, however, is perceived as the norm and it is vital that we support those who choose not to drink and support and promote 'non-drinking' as a valid and socially acceptable choice.

HOW MANY YOUNG PEOPLE CHOOSE NOT TO DRINK ALCOHOL OR USE OTHER DRUGS?

Alcohol and other drug use continues to be regarded by young people as a major issue. In a recent survey of more than 20 000 young Australians aged between fifteen and nineteen, when asked to identify the three issues that they considered to be the most important from a national perspective, alcohol and other drugs was rated highest (equity and discrimination, and mental health being the other two of most concern).[1]

At the same time we are seeing growing numbers of young people choosing not to drink alcohol. The latest Australian Secondary School Alcohol and Drug (ASSAD) Survey found that the proportion of twelve- to seventeen-year-olds who reported never consuming alcohol had risen from 11 per cent in 1999 to 32 per cent in 2014.[2] The number of students who classified themselves as a 'non-drinker' had increased across all age groups between 2011 and 2014. The most significant rise was among fifteen-year-olds, with 70 per cent reporting being a 'non-drinker' in 2014 compared to 59 per cent in the previous survey. It also found that the number of twelve- to fifteen-year-olds drinking has been decreasing since hitting a peak in 2002, and in 2014 was at its lowest point since the survey began. Although there is concern that illicit drug use is increasing, according to the latest research, use of these substances (other than cannabis) among secondary school students continues to be uncommon.

Due to low levels of use and widespread community support for 'non-use' of illicit drugs, the rest of this chapter will focus primarily on alcohol and supporting 'non-drinking'.

WHY DO THEY MAKE THESE CHOICES?

There has been very little research conducted on those young people who choose not to drink and the reasons behind their decision. The majority of studies in this area have focused on how this group deals with the difficulties of non-drinking at a time in their lives when alcohol consumption is portrayed as the norm and is particularly prominent, often highlighting some of the strategies that non-drinkers use in social situations. It would appear, however, that as more young people make the decision not to drink (or, at the very least, delay their first drink or drink less), more research is being conducted, particularly in university or college settings and, as a result, we are learning more about their motivations.

Some of the more often quoted reasons for young people not drinking include the following:

- Religious and/or cultural prohibitions.
- Sporting or academic ambitions.
- Family history of alcohol misuse.

- Not liking the taste and/or effects of alcohol.
- Cost of alcohol.

In more recent research, some of these continue to be identified as playing a part in a non-drinker's decision (e.g. taste, cost, negative past personal experiences and not fitting in with other commitments); however, on closer examination it would appear the strongest messages and influences on choosing not to drink alcohol come from real-life observations. In a study looking at young people who drink little or no alcohol,[3] in addition to some of those reasons already mentioned, the following influences were identified:

- **Good parental models** – their family set boundaries around appropriate drinking behaviours and had provided them with positive role models in 'how to drink'.
- **Seeing negative effects of alcohol on family members** – as much as the family can provide good role models around sensible drinking, some young people experience the negative consequences of parents' or other family members' alcohol use and the problems it causes to their lives and relationships, leading them to choose to abstain.
- **Seeing negative effects of alcohol on friends and others around them** – friends and others drinking to excess and experiencing problems (e.g. personal harm and damaged social reputations) reinforced the decision not to drink.

WHAT ARE SOME OF THE CHALLENGES THAT THESE YOUNG PEOPLE FACE?

The adolescent years are all about learning where you fit in the world and young people quickly work out what will get them accepted within a peer group and what will find them out on their ear. Although growing numbers of young people are choosing not to drink alcohol, or to drink very little, 'non-drinking' is still perceived as being outside the 'norm'. Going to parties and drinking alcohol is simply a part of what many teenagers do every weekend and those young people who decide that it is not for them often have to suffer the consequences. They have to defend the choices they have made and, as a result, can end up feeling uncomfortable and socially isolated. This is clearly illustrated in the following comment made by a Year eleven girl:

I'm starting to go to a lot of eighteenth birthdays now and I'm increasingly being asked if I want a drink, not only by my friends but by people I don't necessarily know and even the parents of my friends! It's been really easy to simply say I don't drink and leave it at that up to now – I've never really been questioned about my choices before this year – but it's now getting really hard and very annoying! I have no desire to tell people, sometimes complete strangers, my life story – it's not their business why I don't drink but sometimes they just won't let you go with a 'No thank you' – they want to know more. You said you didn't drink – how do you do it? What do you say to people to explain your choice not to drink alcohol?

Any young person who chooses not to drink and then makes it clear to their friendship group and everybody else that that is their decision needs to be fairly resilient. It is difficult to be an adult non-drinker in this country, with few, if any, social gatherings or events where the presence of alcohol is not front and centre. Constantly explaining and often defending the reasoning behind your decision can get tiresome at best. If adults feel that great social pressure, how difficult must it feel for a fifteen- or sixteen-year-old adolescent who is struggling to work out where they fit in the world?

In a culture where drinking is perceived as the norm, it becomes necessary for a young person who doesn't drink to come up with a strategy to explain their non-drinking and still 'save face'. A New Zealand study of final year high school students[4] identified four alternative discourses young non-drinkers used to battle drinking norms:

- **Have legitimate alternative subject positions**
  - 'sporty' and 'healthy' lifestyles
  - religious and/or cultural reasons
- **Construct oppositional leisure identities**
  - rejecting association between 'having fun' and drinking alcohol
  - finding alternative activities
- **Reconstitute alcohol consumption as abject**
  - view alcohol in 'loathsome' terms, thus validating their decision not to drink
- **'Pass as a drinker'**
  - while others hold visible or overt positions as non-drinkers, some attempt to 'pass as a drinker' by holding a bottle or glass and/or acting intoxicated.

The authors commented that 'if the "choice" is between being "okay" or "normal" and being "weird"' it does not seem surprising that many teenagers do conform to the norm of alcohol consumption. In fact, it's surprising that many don't – and growing numbers are choosing not to.

The social pressure that people face around alcohol has been acknowledged by the World Health Organization (WHO) and one of the guiding principles of their Global Alcohol Strategy (2010) is as follows: 'Children, teenagers and adults who choose not to drink alcohol beverages have the right to be supported in their non-drinking behaviour and protected from pressures to drink.'

So how do we best support our young people in this area? Regardless of the evidence, we continue to see 'underage drinking' or teen 'binge drinking' portrayed as the norm by the media and the wider community. This focus reinforces the belief that all young people do or will drink alcohol and creates great problems for those teens who have made the decision to be a non-drinker. It is vital that we attempt to redress the imbalance and start to represent and promote the diversity of young people in relation to alcohol. This is best done by challenging existing stereotypes around underage drinking across all areas of practice (e.g. health and education) and, most importantly, within the family.

WHAT CAN PARENTS DO TO SUPPORT THEIR CHILD IN THEIR DECISION?

Unfortunately, many parents believe that they can do little to influence their child's drinking behaviour. As already discussed, many believe that drinking and getting drunk occasionally is a phase that all teenagers go through and that it is simply a rite of passage into adulthood. This is not true. Increasing numbers of young people are choosing not to drink alcohol and sending the message that to do so is potentially dangerous. Parents can make a real difference in this area and help to redress the imbalance by promoting non-drinking as a valid and socially acceptable option by doing the following:

- **Acknowledge all types of drinking – 'risky', 'moderate' and 'non-drinking'.** There are basically three options that a young person (or anyone for that matter) has when it comes to alcohol. They can choose to drink to excess, drink as responsibly as they are able (acknowledging that there may be a slip-up here and there) or choose not to drink at all. All are valid choices (with varying degrees of risk) and all should be acknowledged. Assuming that every young person will drink alcohol at some point or another is simply not true and can make your child feel something is wrong with them or their choice if that is the path they want to follow.
- **If you know a 'non-drinker' – talk about them!** If you or your partner don't drink alcohol, talk about your decision. You don't need to jam it down your child's throat but if the topic arises, grab the opportunity. If alcohol is a part of your life, a relative or family friend can be wheeled out occasionally to talk about their decisions around drinking with your teens. Your child needs to be aware that adults can have a good time without alcohol and that if they choose not to drink they will

not be a social outcast. It's the least a parent can do for their child, who has made this tough decision.

- **Discuss reasons people choose not to drink** – we know most drink to socialise, so why do people choose not to? This is an important conversation to have with a child, acknowledging different religious and cultural differences, as well as the fact that some people experience great problems with alcohol. Talking to a non-drinker about the reasons they have made their decision is particularly helpful.

- **Promote positive norms** – make sure you 'flip the figures' whenever you get the opportunity. You can almost guarantee that, regardless of the issue, the media will focus on the negative, i.e. how many young people drink. Taking those numbers and flipping them over can be really helpful in showing teens that the majority are not usually doing these things, e.g. most fifteen-year-olds classify themselves as non-drinkers.

- **Challenge misconceptions and avoid generalisations** – alcohol is a drug, not everyone does it, and you can celebrate without it! All too often parents will make huge statements like 'everyone drinks' or 'they will all drink at some time or another', or an even bigger cop-out: 'They're just doing what we did!' Outrageous statements like these are often made to justify bad parenting – they don't really have the time or energy to fight with their teen about rules and boundaries around alcohol, so these types of throwaway lines justify that there wasn't any point in trying to stop them drinking anyway.

- **Be a positive role model** – a child learns so much about alcohol from watching their parents and their drinking behaviour, not only during their teen years but from the very early years. If a parent has a brown paper bag with a couple of bottles in it under their arm every time they go out to socialise with friends, they are sending a very strong message to their children about the role alcohol plays in socialising. Does this mean parents should stop drinking or try to hide their drinking from their child? Of course not – it's just important that adult drinking behaviour is discussed with your teen. Once again, it is also vital to discuss the three options for drinking – ensuring that 'non-drinking' is highlighted as a perfectly valid option.

WHAT CAN PARENTS DO TO BE BETTER ROLE MODELS AROUND ALCOHOL?

Parents are a powerful influence, even during adolescence. Here are some simple things that parents can do that can make a positive impact on your teen's attitudes around alcohol and socialising:

- **Talk about your alcohol use** – how do you try to drink safely?
- **Try to limit your alcohol use** in front of your children.
- **Organise events with families and friends that don't involve alcohol.**
- **Provide food and non-alcoholic beverages** if making alcohol available to guests.
- **Don't portray alcohol as a good way to deal with stress**, e.g. 'I've had a bad day, I need a drink!'
- Sometimes **decline the offer of alcohol.**

IF A YOUNG PERSON HAS MADE THE CHOICE NOT TO DRINK ALCOHOL, WHAT CAN A PARENT DO TO BEST SUPPORT THAT DECISION?

For most parents, having a teen who has elected not to drink, for whatever reason, would be regarded as a blessing and they would be extremely pleased with their child's decision. Sadly, due to the role alcohol plays in our society, there are those parents who worry that if their teen doesn't drink they may find themselves socially excluded. Parties and gatherings play a significant role in the social life of teenagers and experimenting with alcohol is often central to that experience. No parent wants to see their child 'left out' or even bullied because of the decisions they make, but it is vital that parents support their child if they choose not to drink alcohol and acknowledge that it is possible to be a non-drinker and still have a fulfilling social life.

If your teen has told you they are a non-drinker, make sure you take the time to do the following:

- **Congratulate them** – don't make too big a deal out of it but let them know you're proud of their healthy choice.
- **Acknowledge that it can be difficult** – even though there are growing numbers of non-drinkers, they are going to be faced with the alcohol issue at almost every social event they attend. Let them know that it can be very tiring to have to continually explain your decision not to drink and it is likely that there will be both peer and social pressure to 'just have one drink' for the rest of their life.
- **Ask how you can support them** – do they need your help in any way? Are they having any issues with friends? Do they need help with 'outs', i.e. do they need help in coming up with an excuse for not drinking?

HOW SHOULD PARENTS HANDLE THE 'OUT' DISCUSSION?

It is important to remember that not all teenagers need an 'out'. Some young people are strong and confident enough to simply say no, if that is indeed what they want to do. We can provide young people skills in how to say no but for many this can be extremely difficult to put into practice, particularly in regards to alcohol use, and it is important that they have some other sort of strategy in place to assist them when they find themselves in difficult situations.

Talk through options that could cover a range of different ways of saying no, including excuses and delaying or putting off the situation. Even though school-based drug education affords young people the opportunity to discuss and develop such skills and strategies, a parent who has a good relationship with his or her child is able to do this far more effectively. Realistically, how can a student discuss 'outs' in the classroom without letting everyone else know what their strategy is going to be? It just doesn't work. This is something that has to be done in the home.

'OUTS' THAT TEENS CAN USE TO HELP THEM 'SAVE FACE' IF THEY DON'T WANT TO DRINK

- 'I am allergic to alcohol.'
- 'The medication I'm on at the moment doesn't mix well with alcohol.'
- 'I'd love to smoke but I have an uncle with a mental health problem.' (A very popular one for getting out of smoking cannabis.)
- 'I got really drunk last week and I'm trying to have a few weeks off.'
- 'Dad found out I was drinking last weekend and I'll be grounded if I get caught again.'
- 'We've got a big game next week and I'm trying to be as prepared as possible.'
- 'Mum's picking me up this evening and she always checks my breath when I get in the car.'

The best way to do this is to find the right time to approach your child. Conversations in the car can be very positive (they can't get away and they don't have to look at you!) but wherever the discussion takes place, find a time where it is just you and your child and there is no likelihood of an interruption.

Ask them if they have ever been in a situation with their friends which they found difficult or uncomfortable. Offer them an example from your life, making it clear that adults experience this problem as well as teenagers. Talk about peer and social pressure, and maybe discuss some of the things that you do to help you through difficult situations. Offer them your help in coming up with practical strategies to assist them in these situations. If now is not the 'right time', let them know that they can come to you at any time and you will try to help them. Working together to come up with an 'out' strategy has worked for many parents and their teenage children.

> ## DECIDE ON AN 'OUT' WORD
>
> This is a word only to be used by a child when they want help to get out of a situation quickly and still 'save face'. Things to consider when deciding on an 'out' word include:
>
> - Discussion about an 'out' word should be had prior to their teens – establish this early and it's more likely to be used.
> - Choose a word that is unlikely to be used in other contexts but is not going to look unusual or draw unwanted attention when used.
> - A person's name works well (a teen could tell their friends it's a relative), although a number is often used (their parent has requested a code for an appliance).
> - The word or number should be able to be used in either a text (when they are at a party and they want to leave) or in conversation (they're in the car with their friends and they've been asked by them to do something they don't want to do).

HOW CAN THOSE WHO WORK WITH YOUNG PEOPLE SUPPORT THOSE WHO CHOOSE NOT TO DRINK?

Although family, particularly parents, play the most important role in this area and have the greatest influence in shaping a child's attitudes and values around alcohol, it is important to acknowledge the impact of all those who work, or come into contact, with young people also have in this area. Once again, however, whether it's in a school setting or government or community-based agency, the focus continues to be on those who do drink, particularly those who drink to excess. In fact, research has noted that non-drinkers are often 'rendered invisible'[5] by most health promotion and educational strategies due to our obsession with the dominant group of those who do drink.

Of course, there are legitimate reasons for this (e.g. drinkers are usually those with the greatest problems and more likely to need assistance from workers with particular expertise), but continuing to only acknowledge this group is problematic.

Research has also found that young people feel that alcohol education and alcohol messages more broadly are based on the assumption that young people will drink. Non-drinkers interviewed in many of the studies that have been conducted emphasise the importance of presenting not drinking as a legitimate option to young people, parents and society more broadly. In their study of young people who drink little or no alcohol, the authors used the following quote from a female non-drinker about her experience in high school to illustrate this point to those who work with young people, particularly teachers:

> All teachers were telling us okay don't drink this much because this and this happens, *but no one told me that it's okay to not drink*. So I think that could be a very important part for example in high school and at that age to hear that it's okay not to be part of the rest . . .[6]

Here are some simple tips for teachers and others who work with young people to consider when talking about alcohol, which can help support those who choose not to drink:

- **Ensure that every conversation you have around alcohol begins with 'If you choose to drink alcohol . . .' and not 'When you drink alcohol . . .'** Those few words at the beginning of the sentence can make all the difference for those teens who choose not to drink. They make them feel included in the discussion (something that non-drinkers rarely feel in this area), they validate their choices (they have been acknowledged) and build resilience (they're more likely to feel connected).
- **Promote positive norms** – this can be particularly difficult for those who work with 'high-risk' young people, where

drinking is the norm. That said, even in areas where most teens are drinking, it is important that they are made aware that the prevalence of non-drinking is increasing and that, if they choose not to drink, they are not alone.

- **Avoid perpetuation of stereotypes and challenge misconceptions** – workers should be mindful of using stereotypes such as 'all teens binge drink' when speaking to teens as well as to others they work with. These stereotypes reinforce inaccurate perceptions of young people and make those who don't drink feel isolated. If young people make inaccurate statements, challenge them – ask them where they got their information from and correct it when appropriate.

- **Examine your school's/agency's or other organisation's practices around alcohol and drinking** – is alcohol a central part of your fundraising or socialising activities? If it is, ensure that these are discussed and that non-drinking options are also offered when appropriate.

CONCLUSION

This chapter is certainly not about promoting abstinence when it comes to alcohol. We live in a society where alcohol is used widely with the majority of adults drinking reasonably and responsibly. Unfortunately, due to alcohol's popularity and the role it plays in so many people's lives, we tend to only ever talk about two options when it comes to drinking – 'responsible drinking' and 'risky drinking'. There is a third – 'not drinking at all'. This option is rarely discussed and, when it is, is often seen as being related to some kind of problem or personal issue that the person may have. Most adults actively support, both by their actions and by what they say, those teens who choose not to use illicit drugs. The same cannot be said when it comes to alcohol. If our children choose not to drink alcohol, they need to be supported in that choice and the best way to do that is to make it very clear that choosing not to drink is socially acceptable and those who don't drink do not have three heads and are completely normal!

It would be great if we eventually have a society where when someone declines a drink of alcohol, there are no questions about why that choice is made. Unfortunately, we're not there yet.

Author biography

Paul Dillon has been working in the area of drug education for the past twenty-five years. Through his own business, Drug and Alcohol Research and Training Australia (DARTA), he has been contracted by many agencies and organisations across Australia to give regular updates on current drug trends within the community. He continues to work with many school communities to ensure that they have access to good quality information and best practice drug education.

www.darta.net.au

See also:
Chapter 9: Talking About Alcohol and Drugs
Chapter 11: Teens, Parties and Alcohol: A Practical Guide to Keeping Them Safe

11. TEENS, PARTIES AND ALCOHOL: A PRACTICAL GUIDE TO KEEPING THEM SAFE

Paul Dillon

Teenage parties provide young people with valuable opportunities to develop a range of social skills that they need to relate effectively with their peers. As they get older, alcohol is likely to become a part of these social gatherings and, unfortunately, things can go wrong. With safety in mind, this chapter provides some practical tips for those parents planning to host a teenage party, as well as others considering allowing their teen to attend such an event.

INTRODUCTION

Adolescence is a time when young people are likely to start spending far more time with their friends and peers than with their families. This is the stage in their life when they start to develop their own identity, attempting to make it distinct from their parents' and, at the same time, peers, and their views on almost everything start to become increasingly important.

Teenage parties (or 'gatherings', as they are now also called) play an important role in an adolescent's development as they provide opportunities for young people to learn personal and social skills they need as they become adults. The socialising that takes place at parties assists adolescents to strengthen existing friendships and make new ones, as well as to gain all-important peer acceptance. When they are involved in the hosting of these events it also gives them the opportunity to learn the skills of planning and entertaining, and introduces their friends to their parents and other family members.

Most of us remember going to parties on Saturday nights when we were in our teens. It was the place where we had fun with our friends, met new people and, for many, it was where we spent time with our boyfriend/girlfriend in a safe environment. We needed parties and our kids need them as well, if for no other reason than they provide valuable opportunities for young people to socialise in a different environment to that of school.

While teenagers are usually excited by the prospect of a forthcoming party, parents can feel at best stressed and anxious and at worst terrified. Much of their concern is around keeping their children safe and many of their fears are based on media stories of teenage parties 'gone wrong'. Footage of 'out-of-control' parties with hundreds of young people spilling out on to the street, bottles being thrown and police seemingly unable to deal with the situation can often be seen in news coverage across the country. It is important to remember, however, that these are not the norm and that is why they have attracted media attention. There are hundreds of teenage parties held every weekend that run smoothly without any issues at all. Sadly, they are never talked about in the media and, as a result, most parents are now reluctant to host these events and many are also fearful of their teen attending.

Certainly, things can go wrong at teenage parties, particularly when alcohol is involved. Some parties and gatherings do get out of control and tragedies do occur. That said, it is important that these events take place and, when appropriate, that parents permit their children to attend them. The best way to ensure the safety of all involved is for parents to be well informed and plan ahead. With that in mind, this chapter has two parts. The first highlights some important things parents should consider if they are planning to host a teenage party. The second will identify some simple strategies for those parents who are considering allowing their child to attend such an event, to help ensure their child's safety.

TIPS FOR THOSE WHO ARE PLANNING
TO HOST A TEENAGE PARTY

Holding a party for teenagers, whether it is at your home or somewhere you have hired for the evening, is a huge responsibility. Parents planning to host a party for teenagers are providing an environment for a group of young people to get together and have a good time. You need to think about all the possible risks and put things into place to make sure that the party is as safe as possible – for the people coming to the party, your neighbours, and you and your family. Of course, there are no guarantees. No matter what safeguards you put in place, there is always the possibility that something could go wrong. However, the greater the planning, the more likely it is that things will run smoothly. Like anything, put a little effort into the organisation and you are likely to reap rewards in the long term.

Hosting a teenage party can be a great opportunity for you to strengthen your relationship with your child, get to know their friends and become more involved in their life. As such, it is important that **you involve your child in the planning of the party**. You can guarantee that they will have a long list of requirements for what makes a successful evening and together you will need to make many decisions about a wide range of issues, including the provision of alcohol. As much as it is important to have your child's input so that the party can be successful, it is also helpful for your child to be aware of all the planning and hard work that needs to be done to ensure that the night runs smoothly. Your child is then much more likely to appreciate the efforts that have been made by all involved and work cooperatively to resolve challenging issues. As much as your child will benefit from the socialising aspect of attending a party with their friends, they will also learn a great deal by helping put an event together.

Some of the decisions that should be made with your child include the following:

- **What food will be available?** Food is incredibly important to have at any party, particularly if alcohol is going to be served.

It slows down the amount of alcohol people drink but you need to be very careful about having too much salty food, which could make people more thirsty and then likely to drink more. Your child is more likely to know what food is 'socially acceptable' to the current generation of young people and will be of great assistance here.

- **Will alcohol be allowed (if there are over-eighteens attending) or 'tolerated' (if not), and who will serve it if it is?** If you do make the decision to serve alcohol, how are you going to deal with the issue of your underage guests, remembering the legal issues around providing alcohol to minors? If a parent contacts you to ask you about alcohol, are you prepared to defend your decision? Does your child understand the risks involved? Is there going to be a 'free-for-all', i.e. are people going to be able to bring their own and then get their own alcohol whenever they want or will there be someone serving alcohol, monitoring how much people are drinking?

- **If you decide on an alcohol-free party, how will you handle guests who turn up with alcohol?** Your child will undoubtedly not want to be embarrassed by one of their parents taking alcohol off their friends if they arrive with a bottle. If a decision to make a party alcohol-free is made, then a solution to this sort of problem needs to be negotiated carefully beforehand. Simply turning a guest away from the party is not a good option. You do not know whether the young person has been dropped off at your home by their parent or how they're getting home – maybe the parent is returning in a few hours. Sending the young person off into the night with a bottle of something is irresponsible and dangerous. Discuss this with your teenager and see if you can come up with some ideas for dealing with this problem together.

- **How will you handle gatecrashers?** Gatecrashers are now a fact of life at teenage parties, particularly if you are providing alcohol. In the age of social media, mobile phones and texting, it doesn't take long for the word to get out that there is a party happening and that it is the place to be. Will you be handing out invitations to those people who you want to come or will you have a guest list? Will you be hiring security to manage the party or do you have a couple of burly relatives who can handle a difficult situation? What responsibility will your teenager have in looking after the door, particularly considering that they are more likely to know who was invited and who wasn't?

- **What will you do in an emergency?** Organisers of the best-planned parties can end up finding themselves trying to handle an emergency of some description. This does not have to be related to alcohol – when a group of people get together, no matter what their age, things can go wrong. Who will be the person to take responsibility should something go wrong? Who will make the list of emergency numbers and where will it be kept? Discuss with your teenager the necessity of registering your party with the local police and why it is so important. When you do register your party, make sure you do it with your child so that they can see and understand the process.

- **How will the guests be getting home and what time will the party finish?** Unbelievably, this is one aspect of hosting a teenage party that many parents forget about. It is undoubtedly one of the most difficult to police but it needs to be discussed with your child so that they understand the huge responsibility you have taken on. There is no way that you are able to know how each and every guest attending the party is getting home, but if something happens to any of those young people when they leave your home, particularly if they have been drinking, it would be difficult to live with yourself. Stress the importance of having a strict finishing time for the party and advertise that time widely. This will ensure that as many parents as possible know the time and are aware that after that time their children will be asked to leave your home. Hopefully this will reduce the number of teenagers spilling out onto the street and into the parks and other public spaces in your local area after the party has finished.

Most 'successful' parties, particularly for those aged fifteen to sixteen years, that do not experience significant issues are those where a decision has been made not to serve alcohol to those attending and not to tolerate any alcohol being brought into the event. Once that decision has been made and the young person has understood and accepted it, the night is usually successful and runs without incident. It is also important to remember that those whose only intent is to get as drunk as possible usually have no interest in attending those gatherings where they know alcohol rules will be policed.

There is no handbook on how to be the perfect parent; you can only do the best you can do at the time. The same is true when it comes to holding an incident-free teenage party. There are some guidelines that you can follow, some of which have been outlined. Without doubt the best thing you can do to reduce risk is to make the event alcohol free. If a parent believes that this is not an option for their child at their stage of development, they need to ensure they take every precaution to keep the party as safe as possible for all concerned.

TIPS FOR THOSE CONSIDERING ALLOWING THEIR CHILD TO ATTEND A TEENAGE PARTY

When your child is invited to their first teenage party or gathering and they ask you whether they can attend, you are likely to experience a range of emotions. Many parents will initially be excited for their child and pleased that they have been invited to their first social event, i.e. they are socially accepted. Once that initial excitement has died down, however, it is likely that many will start to think about all the things that could go wrong and how they are going to ensure that their child is as safe as possible.

Firstly, and most importantly, **parents must not allow themselves to be bullied into making a decision about whether their child can attend or not.** If both parents are on the scene, make it clear right from the very start that both parents make decisions around parties and gatherings. Adolescents are extremely clever at setting up one parent against the other and it is vital that they understand that there is a united front on this issue. Make it clear to them by telling your child, 'Don't come to me, don't go to [the other parent] – come to *us*!'

THREE PARENTING RULES FOR TEENAGE PARTIES AND GATHERINGS

- If your child says you 'can't' do something, that means you *must*!
- You make the decision how they get home from the party and picking them up yourself is always the safest option.
- Find out as much as you can about the event and don't just rely on your child for the info.

Of course, it is not possible to make an informed decision about a party without good-quality information, so you need to do your homework and find out as much about the event as possible. When it comes to what parents need to know about a party to ensure their child's safety, here are the four key pieces of information that should be gathered:

- Whose party is it and do you know them and/or their parents?
- Where will the party be held?
- Will the parents be there and will they be supervising the party?
- What time does it start and what time does it finish?

Based on the answers to these questions, parents should be able to establish whether or not they think the event is safe for their child to attend or not. This information should be collected regardless of the child's age – it doesn't matter if they're six or sixteen – and if they're invited to anyone's home for a party, doesn't every parent want to know the answer to these questions? Unfortunately, some of the information you will need to make a decision can be difficult to collect, particularly as your child gets older, but it is imperative that you know what type of event they want to attend.

Ask your child questions about the party and where it is being held. Get as much information as you can but it is important that you don't just rely on what your child is willing and able to tell you. Even though you may have the most trusting and open relationship with them, they are unlikely to give you the 'whole story'. This does not mean that they would necessarily lie to you – it's just that, in many cases, they really wouldn't know themselves. As a parent you need to go to the source, i.e. the parents holding the event.

WHERE PARENTS CAN GO FOR INFORMATION ABOUT A PARTY

If your child has been invited to a party, these are the places you can go for information:

- **Ask your child.**
- Go to the source: **contact the parents hosting the party.**
- **Talk to other parents.**
- Look at **social media.**

Most teens will not want their parents making contact with other parents who are hosting parties, and if you've never done this before and you start doing it when they are fifteen years old there are likely to be tantrums. However, if your child knows at the age of ten that you call the house beforehand and you continue to do it over time – it's just what you do – you're not going to have anywhere near as much of an issue in later years. It is also important to note that these calls don't always go well (particularly if you start asking questions about alcohol) and can end up leaving some parents feeling very frustrated, but as far as the safety of your child is concerned, they're vital.

Before you make the call, carefully plan and write down the questions you want to ask the host parents. Questions are going to vary, depending on the age of the child and your own personal values, but essentially they should cover issues such as start and finish times, supervision details and whether alcohol will be permitted or tolerated. Please note the words 'permitted' and 'tolerated', and not 'provided'. Many parents find themselves caught out in this area when they believe they have done their homework and asked all the right questions and are sending their child to an alcohol-free party, when in actual fact, although the host parents don't necessarily provide alcohol they may allow teens to bring their own, or at the very least turn a blind eye to them bringing it in.

QUESTIONS TO ASK HOST PARENTS

Asking parents hosting a party how they are going to handle the alcohol issue is going to be much more difficult. Some of the questions that could be asked include the following:

- How are you going to handle the alcohol issue?
- Is alcohol going to be permitted or tolerated at the party?
- Will an effort be made to stop alcohol being taken into the party?
- Will you be allowing BYO?
- Will there be security?

Talk to other parents as well and find out what they know about the party. What time are you dropping off your child? Where are you dropping them off? Do you know the parents who are putting on the party? Does their information match what you've been told by your son or daughter? This source of information is particularly important if you have concerns about the event, e.g. you called the house and you didn't feel entirely comfortable with the response you got from the parent but you haven't got any concrete reason not to allow your teen to attend. Another option is to look at social media and see what has been posted about the party. If you're doing your due diligence and monitoring your child's online activity to some extent, this should not be too difficult to access and can prove very useful.

Once a decision has been made that your teen can attend, the most important thing a parent needs to plan with their child is how they're going to get there and how they're going to get home. Without a doubt the most important thing to remember here is that **you make these decisions and that taking them and picking**

them up yourself is always the safest option. Of course, it is not always going to be possible (for whatever reason) for parents to get into their car on a Saturday night and drop their child off and/or pick them up. Most parents will need to hand over this responsibility to someone else at some point, and as they get older your teen will put forward other options for getting home and a decision will need to be made as to whether that is acceptable or not. But if you can do it, it is the best option.

When parents are actively involved with getting their teens to and from a party, it provides a range of important opportunities. These include the following:

- **Dropping them off** – this is important because you get to take a look at where they're going, meet the parents hosting the event as well as your child's friends, and make a quick assessment of what type of event it is and whether there are any issues that concern you.
- **Picking them up** – this provides you with so much information about what they've been doing, who they've been with, what the party was like and what actually went down. If you are one of those parents who do make the effort to pick up their child, you're likely to be asked to drive other partygoers home, giving you the opportunity to talk to others who attended the event and potentially strengthen the relationship you have with not only your own child but his or her friends as well. Most importantly, though, you get to ensure that they're safe! There are so many things that can go wrong at a teenage party, but there are so many more that can happen on the way home, particularly if your child or their friends have been drinking.

It is important, however, that parents don't risk jeopardising the positive relationship they have with their teen by obsessing in this area. In their final years of high school when they're not far short of eighteen, calling parents hosting parties to find out about each and every event your teen is invited to would be a recipe for disaster. Of course, if there is a party you are particularly worried about, for whatever reason, do your parental duty and call the hosts and, if need be, try your best to prevent your child from going, but at that age if you push too hard you run the risk of embarrassing your child and damaging your relationship. They are teenagers and they will make mistakes and poor decisions and, as hard as it may be, you have to let them stumble and fall occasionally. That said, you don't do this when they're fourteen or fifteen – it's simply too dangerous and they don't have the life experience should something go wrong. It's at this age when you do your very best to find out all you can about where they'll be on Saturday night, who they're with and when they'll be home.

CONCLUSION

It will be impossible for any parents to know everything about a party that their child attends, regardless of how much effort they put into finding out, and no one can expect a parent to drop off or pick up their teen from every party they attend throughout adolescence. Parents can only do the best they can do at the time.

FIVE SIMPLE TIPS FOR PARENTS AROUND PARTIES AND GATHERINGS

They're certainly not always going to be easy to do, but when it comes to a teen's safety, they are vital:

- **Know where your child is and who they're with** – to make absolutely sure, always take them to where they're going and pick them up. Don't leave it up to someone else to do if you can possibly help it.
- **Always call the parents who are hosting the party or gathering**. Speak to them and find out some basic information about supervision and whether alcohol will be provided or tolerated. Your teen is not going to like this but if something goes wrong and you didn't make that call, you will never forgive yourself.

- **Create rules around parties and gatherings early**, preferably before they start to be invited to these events. Try to make the rules the first time they're invited to a party and you're going to meet lots of resistance – every parent should have rules in this area by the time their child is twelve.
- **Make the consequences of breaking the rules clear and stick to them**, but ensure they understand all rules are made because you love them and want them to be safe.
- **If kids don't like the rules, then they're most probably perfect**. But remember, reward good behaviour and modify the rules as they get older to make sure they're age appropriate.

If you decide to host a teenage party or let your child attend a gathering that they have been invited to, be aware that there is no way you can be prepared for all of the possible scenarios that may occur. It is vital, however, that you realise things can go wrong and do your best to outline some possible strategies that could keep your child and their friends safe should they find themselves in potentially dangerous situations, e.g. if something goes wrong, call 999 or 112. It is extremely important to have this discussion with your child and, most importantly, let them know that they can contact you and you will be there for them, no matter what.

Author biography

Paul Dillon has been working in the area of drug education for the past twenty-five years. Through his own business, Drug and Alcohol Research and Training Australia (DARTA), he has been contracted by many agencies and organisations across Australia to give regular updates on current drug trends within the community. He continues to work with many school communities to ensure that they have access to good quality information and best practice drug education.

www.darta.net.au

See also:

Chapter 9: Talking About Alcohol and Drugs

Chapter 10: Supporting a Young Person in their Decision Not to Use Alcohol or Other Drugs

For more online resources visit:
generationnext.com.au/handbook

BODY IMAGE AND EATING DISORDERS

Understanding Eating Disorders in Young People   181

Excessive Dieting and Exercise   202

Anorexia Nervosa   217

Bulimia and Binge Eating   233

Bigorexia: Muscle Dysmorphia in Young People   250

Fostering a Positive Body Image   265

12. UNDERSTANDING EATING DISORDERS IN YOUNG PEOPLE

**Dr Tina Peckmezian, Dr Michelle Blanchard
& Danielle Cuthbert**

This chapter will provide an overview of eating disorders in adolescence and young adults. Readers will gain an understanding of what eating disorders are, how to recognise the warning signs and how to support someone with an eating disorder.

INTRODUCTION

Eating disorders are serious mental illnesses that are associated with considerable psychological impairment and distress. While estimates of the incidence of eating disorders vary between countries and studies, there is agreement that eating disorders, disordered eating and body image issues have increased worldwide over the last thirty years. Research shows more than 55 per cent of young Australians are dissatisfied with their body by the age of nine, and more than 56 per cent are trying to control their weight by the age of eleven. Disordered eating and eating disorders are both estimated to affect approximately 8 per cent of the Australian population. Although eating disorders can occur in people of all ages, adolescents and young people are at greatest risk.

WHAT ARE EATING DISORDERS?

There are several feeding and eating disorders that are recognised by the *Diagnostic and Statistical Manual of Mental Disorders*. Among these are the following disorders.

Binge eating disorder: A person with binge eating disorder will repeatedly engage in binge eating episodes, where they eat a large amount of food in a short period of time. During these episodes they will feel a loss of control over their eating and may not be able to stop even if they want to. People with binge eating disorder often feel guilty, ashamed, embarrassed or depressed about the amount and the way they eat during a binge eating episode. Unlike bulimia nervosa, individuals with binge eating disorder do not use compensatory behaviours after a binge eating episode. Binge eating disorder is estimated to affect approximately 6 per cent of the Australian population.

Bulimia nervosa: A person with bulimia nervosa will have repeated episodes of binge eating, defined as eating a very large amount of food within a relatively short period of time. This is followed by behaviours that compensate for binge eating episodes as a way of trying to control weight e.g. self-induced vomiting, fasting, excessive exercise or misuse of laxatives, drugs or medications. These behaviours are often concealed and people with bulimia nervosa can go to great lengths to keep their eating and exercise habits secret. Many people with bulimia nervosa experience weight fluctuations and do not lose weight; they can remain in the healthy weight range, be slightly underweight, or may even gain weight. Bulimia nervosa is estimated to affect approximately 1 per cent of the Australian population.

Anorexia nervosa: A person with anorexia nervosa will place severe restriction on the amount and type of food they consume and will be significantly below what is considered to be a healthy weight. Even when people with anorexia nervosa are underweight they will still possess an intense fear of gaining weight or becoming 'fat' and may have a disturbed view of their own body weight or shape. People with anorexia nervosa may also engage in bingeing (eating an abnormally large amount in a short period of time) or compensatory behaviours (such as self-induced vomiting or the misuse of laxatives or diuretics). Anorexia nervosa is estimated to affect approximately 0.5 per cent of the Australian population.

Other Specified Feeding and Eating Disorders (OSFED): A person may present with many of the symptoms of other eating disorders but not meet the full criteria for that diagnosis. In these cases the disorders may be classified as atypical or low frequency/limited duration, under the overall heading of OSFED. This does not mean that the person has a less serious disorder; like the other eating disorders, OSFED is characterised by severe distress and impairment to quality of life. OSFED is estimated to affect approximately 1.4 per cent of the Australian population.

What are the risk factors for an eating disorder?

The factors that contribute to the onset of an eating disorder are complex. Each person's experience is influenced by a unique mix of biological and environmental factors. Like most health conditions, a combination of several different factors may increase the likelihood that a person will experience an eating disorder at some point in their life. Known contributing risk factors include the following:

Genetic vulnerability: There is evidence that eating disorders have a genetic basis, meaning that certain genes may increase the likelihood of a person developing an eating disorder. This genetic influence results from the complicated interaction between many genes and a myriad of environmental factors. Genetic influences are also associated with certain personality traits and risk factors for eating disorders, such as perfectionism, and these traits may shape the clinical features of an individual's disorder.

Psychological factors: Research into anorexia nervosa and bulimia nervosa specifically has identified a number of personality traits that may be present before, during and after recovery from an eating disorder. These include perfectionism, obsessive-compulsiveness, neuroticism, negative emotionality, harm avoidance and low self-esteem.

Sociocultural influences: Evidence shows that sociocultural influences play a role in the development of eating disorders, particularly among people who internalise the beauty ideal of thinness. Images communicated through mass media such as television, magazines and advertising are often airbrushed and altered to achieve a culturally perceived image of 'perfection' that does not actually exist. In addition, social media platforms now have filters which encourage users to edit photos and alter their appearance.

Protective factors: Opposite to risk factors, protective factors lower the likelihood of an illness-related outcome. These include individual factors such as high self-esteem, positive body image, emotional reasoning and assertiveness, and sociocultural factors, such as eating regular meals with the family, or belonging to cultural and social groups that do not over-emphasise the value of weight and shape.

How to recognise eating disorders

A person with an eating disorder may have disturbed eating behaviours coupled with extreme concerns about weight, shape, eating and body image. Due to the nature of an eating disorder, a person may go to great lengths to hide, disguise or deny their behaviour. They may display a combination of these symptoms:

Physical warning signs

- Rapid weight loss or fluctuation in weight.
- Fainting or dizziness.
- Always feeling tired and not sleeping well.
- Feeling cold most of the time, even in warm weather.
- Loss of or disturbance of menstrual periods in girls and women.

- Swelling around the cheeks or jaw, calluses on knuckles, damage to teeth and bad breath, which can be signs of vomiting.

Psychological warning signs
- Preoccupation with eating, food, body shape and weight.
- Feeling anxious around mealtimes.
- Feeling 'out of control' around food.
- Having a distorted body image.
- Feeling obsessed with body shape, weight and appearance.
- Rigid thoughts about food being 'good' or 'bad', having to eat or exercise at certain times (strict routine).
- Changes in emotional and psychological state (e.g. depression, anxiety, irritability, low self-esteem).
- Using food as a source of comfort (e.g. eating as a way to deal with boredom or depression).
- Using food as self-punishment (e.g. refusing to eat due to stress or other emotional reasons).

Behavioural warning signs
- Dieting behaviour (e.g. fasting, counting calories/kilojoules, avoiding food groups).
- Eating in private and avoiding meals with other people.
- Evidence of binge eating (e.g. disappearance of large amounts of food).
- Changes in clothing style (e.g. wearing baggy clothes).
- Compulsive or excessive exercising (e.g. exercising in bad weather, in spite of sickness, injury or social events; and experiencing distress if exercise is not possible).
- Making lists of good or bad foods.
- Suddenly disliking food they have always enjoyed in the past.
- Obsessive rituals around food preparation and eating that are not culturally sanctioned practices.
- Extreme sensitivity to comments about body shape, weight, eating and exercise habits.

- Secretive behaviour around food (e.g. saying they have eaten when they haven't, hiding uneaten food).
- Avoiding social situations or events.

Having awareness about eating disorders and the warning signs and symptoms can make a marked difference to the severity and duration of the illness. Seeking help at the first warning sign is much more effective than waiting until the illness has advanced.

COMMON MYTHS AND MISCONCEPTIONS ABOUT EATING DISORDERS

Myth: Eating disorders are a lifestyle choice, not a serious illness.

Fact: The truth is that eating disorders are serious mental illnesses; they are not a lifestyle choice or a diet gone 'too far' and people can't 'just stop' their eating disorder. People with eating disorders require treatment for both mental and physical health addressing the underlying psychological and medical issues.

Myth: Eating disorders are a cry for attention or a person 'going through a phase'.

Fact: People with eating disorders are not seeking attention or 'going through a phase'. In fact, due to the nature of these illnesses, a person with an eating disorder may go to great lengths to hide, disguise or deny their behaviour, or may not recognise that there is anything wrong.

Myth: Eating disorders are about vanity.

Fact: Eating disorders are serious and potentially life-threatening mental illnesses, in which a person experiences severe disturbances in eating and exercise behaviours because of distortions in thoughts and emotions, especially those relating to body image or feelings of self-worth. There are genetic and personality vulnerabilities as well as social and environmental triggers. Eating disorders are not just about food or weight, vanity, willpower or control. They are fuelled by distress, anxiety, stress and cultural pressures.

Myth: Families, particularly parents, are to blame for eating disorders.

Fact: A common misconception is that family members can cause eating disorders through their interactions with a person at risk. While there are environmental triggers which may impact on the development and continuation of an eating disorder, there is no evidence that a particular parenting style causes eating disorders. Clinical guidelines encourage the inclusion of families at each stage of treatment for adolescents, from the initial assessment to providing recovery support.

UNDERSTANDING THE STAGES OF CHANGE

There are five stages of change that a person with an eating disorder may go through. Everyone is different, and some people may go back and forth between these stages.

1. Pre-contemplation

In the pre-contemplation stage a person with an eating disorder will most likely be in denial that there is a problem. You might have noticed some of the warning signs and feel concerned about the person, but they will have little or no awareness of the problems associated with their disordered eating. Instead, they may be focused on controlling their eating patterns, and may be hostile, angry or frustrated when approached and may feel unwilling or afraid to let go of these behaviours.

What you can do:

- Show compassion and understanding.
- Stay calm and try to see things from their point of view using active listening techniques.
- Take the focus off their disordered eating by talking about their interests and goals in life.
- Encourage or support access to medical treatment if their health is compromised.

2. Contemplation

A person with an eating disorder in the contemplation stage will have an awareness of their problems and may be considering the benefits of changing some of their behaviours. They swing between wanting to change and wanting to maintain their disordered eating habits.

What you can do:

- Listen to what the person has to say. Demonstrate that you are listening to what they are saying, and that you understand their struggle. You can even say it back to them, e.g. 'I hear you saying that part of you feels like you want to change, while another part of you feels scared of changing . . .'
- If they talk about wanting to change their behaviours, encourage this idea and suggest accessing support to assist with making these changes.

3. Preparation/determination

In this stage the person with the eating disorder has decided they want to change their behaviour and is preparing to make these changes.

What you can do:

- Be informed. Learn as much as you can about the steps you and the person you are caring for need to take in order to recover.
- Work with the person to identify their goals and develop a detailed approach of how you will manage the changes together, including plans for treatment, wellness and crisis support.

4. Action

During the action stage, the person has decided they want to change and will need support to help them take the first steps towards recovery. The person can move backwards and forwards in their development during this stage and relapse can be common.

What you can do:

- Acknowledge how difficult it is to change and recover from an eating disorder.

- Support the person through challenges and let them know you believe in them.
- Review and refine goals and treatment plans as progress is made.

5. Maintenance

In the maintenance stage a person will have changed their behaviour and may be focusing on maintaining their new, healthier habits while learning to live without an eating disorder. This takes time and requires commitment. Relapse is still possible during this stage.

What you can do:

- Work together with the person to identify triggers that may affect their recovery.
- Accept relapse as a part of the process of recovery and put systems and strategies in place to help avoid relapse.
- Show care, patience and compassion.

CASE STUDIES

Case Study 1: Adam is seventeen years old. He has previously been diagonised with depression and he often uses eating as a way to help manage his feelings. At times of stress or frustration, he can't stop himself from overeating. Sometimes Adam is so absorbed with his difficult thoughts and feelings that he does not realise how much he has eaten. Once Adam regains control of these situations he experiences intense feelings of shame and guilt about his weight, the amount of food he has eaten and the manner in which he has eaten it. He is so embarrassed about his eating habits that he avoids eating with others, especially at school.

Case Study 2: Melanie attends the local school and is in Year Nine. She has a reserved, quiet demeanour and maintains few close friendships within and outside school. Melanie is talented academically and musically; however, she has been finding this year at school increasingly difficult.

Over the last four months, she has been observed missing meals at school and avoids eating with others, including her family. She is currently a healthy weight for her age and height, although her weight often fluctuates. Melanie has disordered eating patterns, including participating in fad diets. One of her closest friends is aware that she has high levels of self-loathing and guilt after eating. Her music teacher has expressed concern about her high levels of fatigue, irritability and increasingly impaired concentration.

Would you suspect Adam or Melanie have an eating disorder? When, where and how would you consider supporting and referring them for help?

Given the characteristics and symptoms described, Adam is likely to be living with binge eating disorder, while Melanie is showing signs of disordered eating, which may indicate the presence of an eating disorder. In both cases, it is imperative to intervene early and refer individuals to specialised support services and treatments that are targeted towards eating disorders. More information and resources can be found in the 'Where to get help' and 'Resources' sections at the end of this chapter.

SOCIAL MEDIA: RISKS AND STRATEGIES FOR SAFER USE

Social media plays an increasingly important role in the lives of young people. For many, social media provides an accessible and powerful toolkit for finding information, building relationships and promoting a sense of identity and belonging. For others, online communities can be an unsafe space, and being aware of the risks can help educators and carers take the appropriate precautions to ensure safe use.

- **Social media platforms** allow users to personalise and curate their online presence and instantaneously communicate with peers across a range of handheld devices. Images of thin, attractive men and women are widely available online and expose viewers to unrealistic standards of beauty that can have a detrimental impact on body image.

- **Thinspiration and fitspiration** refer to images of thin and fit individuals that are shared online, generally with the intention of motivating others to a slimmer physique or healthier lifestyle. While some viewers may be inspired by these images to make positive changes, they can also increase body dissatisfaction by leading viewers to compare their own bodies to these images and feel less attractive themselves.

- **'Pro-eating disorders' websites** encourage disordered eating behaviour and provide a social forum for the exchange of photos, tips and support. They often contain advice that directly encourages unhealthy and extreme weight and shape control behaviours, as well as tips on how to best conceal these behaviours. Termed 'pro-ana' when supporting anorexia and 'pro-mia' when supporting bulimia, these sites positively portray the anorexic or bulimic lifestyle and focus on themes of perfection, physical transformation, strength and success.

Strategies for parents, educators and young people

- **Set realistic expectations**: Parents and educators should encourage moderation and conscientious use of social media platforms rather than abstinence.

- **Engage and listen**: Where 'unsafe' use is observed, engage in conversation with the young person to understand their motivations for interacting with the site and what they are taking away from their experience.

- **Be conscientious**: For young people, it is helpful to intentionally follow pages that contain positive content and unfollow pages that contain negative or triggering content, such as pages that consistently portray the thin, digitally enhanced beauty ideal.

- **Take action:** Facebook, Twitter and Instagram all have the option to report individual posts or pages that are problematic.

- **Learn more**: For parents and educators, www.internetmatters.org can be a helpful starting point for information about popular sites and their safety policies. Media literacy interventions are an evidence-based eating disorders prevention strategy that may also be helpful. These interventions teach individuals to critically evaluate the media so that media messages are less persuasive, with the goal of reducing the negative effect that the media has on body satisfaction. Online resources, such as those found on the Beat website (www.beateatingdisorders.org.uk) provide additional information and support.

WHAT CAN FAMILIES AND CARERS DO TO HELP?

Families, carers and support services play a crucial role in the care, support and recovery of people with eating disorders. They can contribute to an effective collaborative care approach in three key areas:

- **Supporting engagement with treatment:** A characteristic of eating disorders is that the person will be reluctant to seek help, often denying illness or concealing behaviours. People in close relationships to the person with an eating disorder play a vital role in influencing help seeking, raising awareness of problem behaviours, and supporting recognition of stages in recovery.
- **Supporting implementation of treatment:** The family or support networks are integral members of the treatment team. Carers require skills and knowledge to support treatment in the context of a dynamic illness that manifests in different ways at different points in its course.
- **Providing long-term care and support:** Long-term treatment requires an equally long-term commitment from the person's support network with implications for the family or carer's economic, social, physical and mental wellbeing.

Tips for carers

The effects of an eating disorder are often felt not only by the person experiencing it, but also by their family and support network. If you are caring for someone with an eating disorder, it is possible that at some point you may feel:

- Distressed about what is happening to you, the person you care for, or your family.
- Burnt out from caring for someone with an eating disorder, on top of existing commitments.
- Guilty about your 'role' in the illness. You may fear that you are in some way responsible.
- Confused about the best way to help, both daily and in the long-term goal of recovery.
- Anxious and afraid about the physical and psychological changes in the person you care for.
- Hopeless or helpless about your ability to provide support.

All of these feelings are normal. Caring for someone with an eating disorder is a huge responsibility and comes with considerable personal strain. You may want to 'fix' the problem and feel frustrated when you can't. You may start to fear and dread mealtimes. You may feel like the eating disorder has taken over your life, leaving no time for the things you used to enjoy as an individual.

Here are some tips to help you cope with the challenges along the way:

- **Learn as much as you can**: Having a good understanding of eating disorders will help you to identify what is happening to the person you are caring for.
- **Remember who the person is:** Do not let the eating disorder take over the person's identity. Try to view the illness as the problem and the person you are caring for as part of the solution.

- **Communicate openly**: Communicate without judgement or negativity, and allow the person to express how they are feeling. Avoid focusing on food and weight and instead try to talk about the feelings that may exist beneath the illness.

- **Stay positive**: Draw attention to the positive attributes the person has. Talk about the things they enjoy and the things you love about them. Reminding the person of their life outside of their illness can help them to realise there is more to them than their eating disorder.

- **Make time for yourself**: Prioritising 'time out' for yourself will help restore your energy. The better you care for yourself, the more you will be able to help the person you are caring for.

- **Be patient:** People with eating disorders can experience a range of different and conflicting emotions all in one day. It is important to be as calm and patient as possible throughout their recovery and remember that there is no quick fix. Recovery takes time and patience.

- **Seek support:** Professional support can reduce the amount of stress you carry and improve your capacity to care for someone with an eating disorder.

Tips for educators

Education professionals can play an instrumental role in delivering positive messaging about body image and healthy eating and exercise behaviours, and reducing the stigma and misconceptions that surround eating disorders. The following steps and considerations may be helpful:

- **Make time for eating disorders prevention programmes**. Prevention programmes are not all equally successful. Advocate for a programme that is developmentally appropriate and evidence-based.

- **Create a safe and respectful classroom environment.** Use a health-promotion approach by focusing on building self-esteem, a balanced approach to nutrition and physical activity and coping skills that promote resilience.
- **Provide support to students in need.** The effects of an eating disorder may limit a student's ability to keep up to date with their work and participate in activities. Schools should develop a strategy to ensure that the student can manage their studies, and a care plan that identifies a primary support person who will communicate with the student and liaise with the student's family and healthcare professionals (if confidentiality permits).
- **Maintain your professional boundaries.** It is important to maintain a normal teacher–student relationship and not become too involved with the student personally.
- **Involve the family whenever possible.** Families are generally in a better position than schools to encourage children and young adults to seek professional help quickly; however, be mindful of your school's guidelines on sharing confidential information.

HOW TO COMMUNICATE

There is no 'right' or 'wrong' way to talk to someone with an eating disorder and different approaches will work for different people.

1. Be prepared

The most important thing you can do is to be prepared and educate yourself as much as possible about eating disorders. The person you care about may be experiencing high levels of anxiety, shame, embarrassment, guilt or denial, or may not recognise that they have an eating problem. It is important to take this into consideration and be prepared to deal with the person if they respond with anger or denial.

2. Choose a caring environment

Any approach needs to be carried out in a caring manner, in an environment that can support open and calm conversation. For example, it can be beneficial to approach the person in an environment where they feel most comfortable and safe, such as at home. Avoid broaching the topic if you are around food or in situations in which either of you is angry, tired or emotional.

3. Use the right language

If you are approaching someone with an eating disorder, you need to take into account their fear of disclosing their behaviours or feelings. Let them know that you care about them and that you want to help them face the problem and support them through every stage of the healing process.

Below are some **helpful tips** when talking to someone you suspect may have an eating disorder:

- Try to use 'I' statements, e.g. 'I care about you' or 'I'm worried about you'.
- Make the person feel comfortable and let them know it is safe to talk to you.
- Encourage them to express how they feel rather than focusing on how you feel.
- Give your loved one time to talk about their feelings – don't rush them through the conversation.
- Listen respectfully and let them know that you won't judge or criticise them.
- Encourage them to seek help and explain that you will be there with them each step of the way.

There are also certain things you should **try to avoid**:

- Avoid putting the focus on food; instead, try talking about how the person is feeling.

- Do not use language that implies blame or that the person is doing something wrong, e.g. 'You are making me worried.' Instead try, 'I am worried about you.'
- Try not to take on the role of a therapist or dominate the conversation. You do not need to have all the answers; it is most important to listen and create a space for the person to talk.
- Avoid manipulative statements, e.g. 'Think about what you are doing to me' or 'If you loved me you would eat properly.' This can make it more difficult for the person to admit to their problem.
- Do not use any threatening statements, e.g. 'If you don't eat right I will punish you.' This can be emotionally harmful and exacerbate the eating problem.

IS RECOVERY POSSIBLE?

Recovery from an eating disorder *is* possible. Recovery involves overcoming physical, mental and emotional barriers in order to restore normal eating habits, thoughts and behaviours. Evidence shows that the sooner you start treatment for an eating disorder, the shorter the recovery process will be. Seeking help at the first warning sign is much more effective than waiting until the illness is established.

There is no set time for recovery and it is not uncommon for the process to slow down, come to a complete halt or encounter relapses. While this may seem frustrating, it can help to remember that with recovery as the ultimate goal, even the setbacks can be a valuable part of the journey. With the appropriate treatment and a high level of personal commitment, recovery from an eating disorder is achievable.

TIPS TO SUPPORT A HEALTHY RECOVERY

- **Support** – Feeling supported will help a person's treatment and recovery. A circle of support will also decrease the isolation often experienced by people with eating disorders.
- **Hope and motivation** – Having a strong sense of hope coupled with the motivation to change eating disorder behaviours is the foundation of recovery.
- **Healthy self-esteem** – Helping the person to remember they are worthwhile will remind them that recovery is worthwhile too.
- **Understanding and expressing your emotions** – It is normal for a person with an eating disorder to feel a range of emotions and it is helpful to acknowledge and express feelings.
- **Acknowledging setbacks** – With the focus on recovery, even taking a step backwards can still be making progress.
- **Coping strategies** – Developing a list of coping strategies that calm them down and help them regulate their emotions can help during stressful or trigger situations.
- **Engaging in activities and interests** – Revisiting the things they enjoyed before the development of their eating disorder will build self-esteem, give purpose and reconnect them with their surrounding world.

Some of the content in this chapter has been adapted from resources previously written by the National Eating Disorders Collaboration (NEDC). For more information or to access evidence-based resources please see www.NEDC.com.au.

WHERE TO GET HELP

If you are in a crisis situation, need immediate medical assistance or are at risk of harming yourself, please contact emergency services by dialling 999 or 112.

Samaritans

Samaritans operates a twenty-four-hour confidential telephone service, offering you a safe place to talk any time you like about whatever's getting to you. You don't have to be suicidal, and the service is available to young people as well as those over eighteen.

Helpline: 116 123 (free)

Hours: Samaritans is available 24/7, 365 days of the year

Email: jo@samaritans.org

Write to: Freepost RSRB-KKBY-CYJK, PO Box 9090, Stirling, FK8 2SA

Childline

Childline operates a twenty-four-hour confidential telephone and online counselling service for anyone under the age of nineteen in the UK.

Helpline: 0800 1111 (free)

Online counselling and email: www.childline.org.uk

Hours: Childline is available 24/7; 365 days of the year

Message boards are available for asking questions and sharing experiences

If you suspect that someone you know has an eating disorder, it is important to seek help immediately. The earlier you seek help the closer you are to recovery.

Beat

Beat is the UK's leading charity supporting those affected by eating disorders and campaigning on their behalf, and provides telephone, email and web support. People with an eating disorder, families, carers, friends and professionals can contact the Helpline for information, personalised support and information on treatment and services.

Helplines (free): Adult 0808 801 0677; Youthline 0808 801 0711.

Helplines are open 365 days of the year, 3 p.m. to 10 p.m.

Email: help@beateatingdisorders.org.uk

Beat Youthline provides email support for anyone under eighteen: fyp@beateatingdisorders.org.uk

Message boards are available, both for adults and for those under eighteen

Website: www.beateatingdisorders.org.uk

Author biography

This chapter was prepared by The Butterfly Foundation for Eating Disorders, drawing on the resources developed by the National Eating Disorders Collaboration (NEDC). The NEDC is funded by the Australian Government Department of Health. The NEDC is a collaboration of people and organisations with expertise in the field of eating disorders, whose primary purpose is to develop a nationally consistent, evidence-based approach to the prevention and management of eating disorders across Australia.

www.NEDC.com.au

www.thebutterflyfoundation.org.au

See also:

Chapter 4: Anxiety in Young People
Chapter 5: Depression in Young People
Chapter 6: Understanding Self-harm
Chapter 13: Excessive Dieting and Exercise
Chapter 14: Anorexia Nervosa
Chapter 15: Bulimia and Binge Eating
Chapter 16: Bigorexia: Muscle Dysmorphia in Young People
Chapter 17: Fostering a Positive Body Image

Recommended websites:

NHS: www.nhs.uk/conditions/Eating disorders
National Centre for Eating Disorders: eating-disorders.org.uk
Anorexia and Bulimia Care: www.anorexiabulimiacare.org.uk
Beat: www.beateatingdisorders.org.uk

Further resources:

Emergency: 999 or 112
Samaritans
    Helpline: 116 123 (free)

Childline
  Helpline: 0800 1111 (free)
Beat
  Adult helpline: 0808 801 0677 (free)
  Youthline: 0800 801 0711 (free)

Further reading:

Hay, P, Chinn, D, Forbes, D, Madden, S, Newton, R, Sugenor, L, Touyz, S, Ward, W 2014, 'Royal Australian and New Zealand College of Psychiatrists Clinical practice guidelines for the treatment of eating disorders', *Australia and New Zealand Journal of Psychiatry*, vol. 48, pp 977–1008.

Mental Health First Aid 2008, 'Eating disorders – First Aid Guidelines', pp 1–5.

NEDC, 2010, *Eating Disorders Prevention, Treatment and Management: An Evidence Review.*

For more online resources visit:
generationnext.com.au/handbook

13. EXCESSIVE DIETING AND EXERCISE

**Amy Burton, Andreea Heriseanu,
Brooke Donnelly & Phillip Aouad**

This chapter will provide an overview of excessive dieting and exercise in adolescents, how to recognise these behaviours, and what to do for support. We will discuss the important difference between 'healthy' changes to diet and exercise and 'excessive' dieting and exercising.

INTRODUCTION

Not all eating disorders can be simply categorised into 'anorexia nervosa', 'bulimia nervosa' or 'binge eating disorder'. A range of problematic eating and weight-loss behaviours can have devastating impacts on individuals and their loved ones. These less-specific types of eating disorders and disordered eating patterns can often go unnoticed, undiagnosed and, consequently, untreated. These behaviours have a tendency to start out as something small and can quickly develop into a full eating disorder. Therefore, it is important to notice the development of excessive dieting and/or exercise and to start to address these problematic behaviours early.

WHY IS THIS IMPORTANT FOR YOUNG PEOPLE?

Eating disorders are known to 'strike' at the very time our bodies and brains are undergoing a critical stage of development: during early to mid adolescence. If eating disorders are left untreated, they will likely have a serious, detrimental effect on the young person. Eating disorders usually develop within the context of dieting and/or excessive exercise. Both of these behaviours are often conducted in secret and are rarely openly discussed by the young person.

We all go through a developmental 'window' in adolescence, where optimal nutrition and sleep are needed in order to reach our genetic potential in terms of physical, brain and emotional development. If we pass through this 'window of development' and don't appropriately nourish ourselves, we miss a vital opportunity that can't be reversed later on.

In sum, it is critical to be aware of excessive dieting and exercise in young people in order to help avoid issues with:

- Physical development, e.g. stunted physical growth such as height; bone health.
- Brain development and functioning, e.g. neural networks required to achieve emotional and social development and functioning may be affected.
- The presentation of significant warning signs for the development, or presence, of eating disorders such as anorexia nervosa, bulimia nervosa and/or body image disturbance.

A 'BALANCED' LIFESTYLE

We know that we need to eat a balanced diet and engage in regular exercise for optimal health. There is a very large and very profitable diet and fitness industry that fills our newspapers, magazines and television programs with advertisements that tell us we need to eat in a certain way or complete a particular exercise in order to be 'healthy'. Often, we get bombarded with conflicting information about what we 'need' to do to be 'healthy'. Therefore, it can be difficult to navigate all of the different messages out there and to work out how to lead a healthy lifestyle, without getting caught up in all of the latest diet fads and exercise crazes. Unfortunately, there is no 'magic pill' that makes someone healthy; it is a combination of factors that lead to optimum health. We are often told that, as a society, we need to eat less and exercise more, but it is certainly not that simple. Like other behaviours, eating and exercise patterns can be placed on a spectrum, where too much or too little has negative consequences on the body. Eating too much or too little can severely affect our body, ranging from the impacts of malnourishment to health complications related to being overweight and obese. The same principle applies to exercise: too little exercise can have implications for cardiovascular health, but too much exercise is also not good for our bodies or our minds. So, what constitutes a healthy diet and a healthy amount of exercise? Well, this differs from person to person, based on a range of factors. Therefore, this chapter aims to help define what health professionals consider to be 'healthy' behaviours and what would be considered 'excessive' and, ultimately, 'not healthy', for young persons.

AUSTRALIAN DIETARY GUIDELINES

In fact, Australian Dietary Guidelines recommend that for optimal health people should eat a 'wide variety of nutritious foods' from all the five major food groups (listed in order from more to less):

1. Grains (including wholegrain cereals, rice, pasta, breads, muesli and oats)
2. Vegetables
3. Meat, seafood, eggs, tofu, nuts, seeds and legumes/beans
4. Dairy (or dairy alternatives)
5. Fruit

Additionally, the Australian Dietary Guidelines also recommend small amounts of oils, and occasional consumption of small amounts of 'treat foods' (those high in sugar, salt, fat or alcohol).
It is also recommended that we drink plenty of water. For information in the UK, visit www.bda.uk.com/foodfacts/home.

Source: National Health and Medical Research Council. (2016). *The Guidelines. Eat For Health*. www.eatforhealth.gov.au/guidelines

A HEALTHY DIET

To best nourish our bodies and our brains, it is important to eat a nutritious diet. This is particularly important for children and adolescents whose bodies and brains are rapidly changing and developing. It's important to eat enough food to meet your energy requirements. Such requirements will vary greatly between individuals, based on an array of influences including, but not limited to, genetics, activity level, age, sex, rate of development and external environmental factors. In order to properly maintain health and meet our energy needs, it is important to eat meals and snacks that include a range of food groups, and it is important to eat regularly throughout the day (often in the form of three meals and two to three snacks, but this can also vary from person to person).

UNHEALTHY DIETING

The previous section describes what is considered by dietitians, nutritionists and other health professionals to be a 'healthy' diet. However, the word 'diet' is often associated with a deliberate change in eating pattern for the purpose of losing weight or influencing body shape.

The concept of 'dieting' is difficult to avoid, with the word being printed on the cover of most women's magazines, and also appearing at an increasing rate on men's magazines. Articles within these magazines describe the latest 'fad diets' that promise rapid weight loss or increased muscle tone. These types of diets usually promote a restriction of total intake of food such that food consumed does not meet the person's energy requirements. These restrictive diets usually require the individual to 'count calories' or to consume smaller portions of food; some even require the person to engage in 'fasting' (i.e. the person can only eat an extremely small amount of food on some days). The other main type of 'fad diets' requires the person to restrict or even completely refrain from eating foods from one of the major food groups – usually carbohydrates, fats or sugars.

Another common type of 'fad diet' encourages the dieter to consume a large amount of a particular type of food, sometimes encouraging the dieter to consume only this one type of food with a promise that the food has specific weight-loss properties. Some examples of foods featured in this type of diet include grapefruit, green tea and protein bars as well as 'detox' diets.

None of these types of fad diets meet the recommendations set by the Australian Dietary Guidelines for optimal health, which states that we should eat a variety of foods from all of the five major food groups, and to eat a sufficient amount to meet our energy requirements.

Although 'dieting' in this way can seem very commonplace in western society, engaging in these 'unhealthy' diets can have very severe consequences leading to poor short-term and/or long-term health outcomes. Examples of known consequences of unhealthy diets include dehydration, malnutrition, vitamin/nutrient deficiencies, electrolyte imbalances, loss of menstrual cycle in women, inhibited physical growth and brain development, muscle atrophy/ wasting, suppressed metabolism, hypertension (high blood pressure) or hypotension (low blood pressure), osteoporosis, osteopenia, gastrointestinal diseases and conditions, and, in some severe cases, major organ and heart failure. In addition to this range of extremely undesirable effects on the body, engaging in unhealthy diets can also have psychological and neurological impacts including poorer cognitive function, difficulties with concentration and learning, more rigid and inflexible thinking styles (i.e. 'black and white', 'good and bad', 'all or nothing' thinking), and even changes in the brain structure and brain chemistry. The good news is that these changes are all reversible with good nutrition (normal, flexible eating) and time.

Given all of the potential negative physical and psychological consequences of dieting, it is clear to see why it is *particularly* dangerous for young people with developing brains and bodies. Sadly, however, it is not uncommon for teenagers (and even children under the age of twelve) to commence a 'diet' for the purpose of losing weight or changing their body shape. For many people, dieting behaviour comes and goes, and does not develop into a more severe condition. However, for some people, dieting behaviour can develop into *disordered eating* in the form of excessive dieting (usually when a person's diet involves strict rules and more extreme behaviours) or a distinct eating disorder such as anorexia nervosa, bulimia nervosa, binge eating disorder or an atypical eating disorder.

Please visit the Generation Next website to read about the evolution of 'the diet'.

EXCESSIVE DIETING AND DISORDERED EATING

A population study found that 20 per cent of Australians aged between fifteen to twenty-four years reported that they are currently on a 'very strict diet' or they are fasting ('eating hardly anything at all for a time') for the purpose of changing their weight or body shape.

There exists a 'slippery slope' between dieting, excessive dieting and disordered eating, and in many cases the boundary between these is unclear. However, in all cases these behaviours and conditions are dangerous, and have very serious physical and mental health implications that are particularly problematic in adolescents. Therefore, there is cause for alarm.

This section will describe types of behaviours and conditions associated with excessive dieting and disordered eating practices.

Orthorexia

Orthorexia is not a recognised eating disorder, but it's a condition that has been receiving more recognition in recent years. Orthorexia is the term used to describe people who have an 'unhealthy' obsession with 'healthy' eating. The individuals experiencing orthorexia often become fixated on what is the 'correct' eating regimen. Orthorexia will often start out as an attempt by the individual to eat more healthily, but over time the person becomes obsessed with their food choices, creating strict rules about what they can and cannot eat. Their self-esteem becomes intertwined with their ability to eat 'correctly', which can sometimes lead to a sense of righteousness and feelings of superiority over others, particularly in relation to food choices and eating. In many cases, orthorexia leads to very restrictive food intake (as few foods will meet their strict criteria for 'correctness') and as a result their health suffers. This condition often ties in with the latest 'fad diets' that promise to lead to optimum health. Recent examples of the types of diets that people with orthorexia become obsessed with include 'clean eating' and the 'paleo' diet. There isn't anything wrong with wishing to make healthy eating choices; however, if someone becomes fixated on 'healthy eating' and is beginning to dedicate a lot of time and attention to their diet, or if they are unable to deviate from their diet rules without experiencing guilt and self-loathing, then this is not actually leading to best health any longer – they are more than likely neglecting other areas of their life and reducing their overall wellbeing.

Other Specified Feeding or Eating Disorder (OSFED)

This disorder applies when eating disorder symptoms are present, which cause distress and reduced functioning but do not meet the full criteria for a diagnosis such as anorexia, bulimia or binge eating disorder. OSFED can include disorders such as:

- Atypical anorexia nervosa, where a person's weight may still be in the 'healthy' range, despite considerable weight loss.
- Atypical bulimia nervosa/binge eating disorder, where a person may still have objective binges and loss of control over eating, but less often than people with bulimia or binge eating disorder do.
- Purging Disorder, where a person may not have binge episodes, but is purging (e.g. vomiting, using laxatives or diuretics) to change their weight or shape.
- Night Eating Syndrome, where someone might eat after waking up from sleep, or may eat an excessive amount after the evening meal, such that they experience distress or decreased function.

Unspecified Feeding or Eating Disorder (UFED)

Similar to OSFED, eating disorder symptoms are present but do not meet the full criteria for another disorder; however, there is not enough information to make a more specific diagnosis.

Avoidant/Restrictive Food Intake Disorder (ARFID)

Formally known as Selective Eating Disorder (SED), ARFID is an eating disorder whereby an individual avoids certain foods based on its appearance, smell, taste, texture, past negative experience or belief that it should not be consumed. While not strictly related to excessive or extreme dieting, it does deserve a mention. It is often seen in 'picky eaters' (especially in young people) who will restrict their intake to avoid foods that they do not like or wish to eat. It should be made clear that ARFID cannot be the result of other neuropsychological or sensory disorders such as Autism Spectrum Disorder (ASD) – also known as Asperger's disorder – it is a psychological aversion to eating or feeding that can lead to weight loss, malnutrition and psychosocial developmental problems.

HEALTHY EXERCISE

People exercise for many reasons: for their health, to feel good or to stop feeling bad, out of habit, to control their shape and/or weight, for social reasons, or to increase physical skills. 'Exercise' includes planned sessions of activity (such as going for a run, attending a class at the gym, or playing sport), but also unstructured, or 'incidental' exercise (such as walking to and from public transport, gardening, cleaning, fidgeting, walking around the shops). Physical activity provides many health benefits, such as strengthening bones and muscles, and reducing the risk of illnesses such as cardiovascular diseases, type 2 diabetes, and other metabolic syndrome-related problems. Exercise is also helpful for mental health, as it can boost mood and reduce anxiety, help relieve stress, improve memory and sleep. While regular, moderate exercise is generally recommended, exercise that is excessive or compulsive can be harmful to both physical and mental health. In determining what is 'healthy' exercise, individual differences need to be considered – what may be appropriate for one individual may be harmful for another – this is why it's important to check which exercise type and level is right for you with a health professional, especially when starting out, or if you have experienced difficulties due to exercise in the past.

EXCESSIVE EXERCISE

The many health benefits of exercise are well known. However, exercise is not always good for someone's health. When exercise becomes compulsive or excessive, it can have a particularly negative effect on health, sometimes causing serious long-term injury. If someone begins exercising too frequently, too intensely, or in a strict and obsessive manner, there is cause for concern for that person's mental health as well as their physical health.

The first type of problematic exercise is *compulsive exercise*; this is sometimes also referred to as an 'exercise addiction'. Compulsive exercise refers to the person's thinking and attitude in relation to their exercise regimen and does not directly refer to the act of exercising itself. The type of exercise that they are engaging in does not necessarily have to be 'excessive' in nature (i.e. the compulsive exercise may be walking ten thousand steps every day); however, the exercise is compulsive if the person feels that they *need* to complete their planned exercise and they find it difficult to decrease frequency, duration or intensity of exercise, or to stop exercising. This type of problematic exercising becomes apparent when the person is unwilling to alter their exercise routine when unwell, when injured, or when they have other commitments (such as school, work or social plans). Compulsive exercise can lead to poor physical health outcomes – these occur when the person continues to exercise when they are sick or injured, or if they continue to increase the duration, frequency or intensity of their exercise. Compulsive exercise also has a negative impact on the person's mental health as the person can become obsessed with their exercise routine (you might feel that the young person's whole life revolves around their exercise plans), they can become socially withdrawn and they can start encountering problems in school or their workplace due to their over-commitment to exercise.

Excessive exercise refers to an amount or type of exercise that is more than what is necessary for the maintenance of good health. The exercise can be excessive in a variety of ways – too frequent, too long in duration or too intense. Just as a 'healthy' amount/type of exercise varies from person to person based on a variety of different reasons, what constitutes an 'unhealthy' amount/type of exercise also varies. What one person might experience as a healthy amount of exercise for their body and fitness level may be an excessive amount of exercise for a different person. The type of exercise doesn't matter – someone could be engaging in an excessive amount of walking, yoga, fitness classes, running or other cardio, or lifting weights. The key differentiating factor that makes something 'excessive' is that the behaviour becomes rigid and inflexible among other commitments in a person's life – often causing distress if it is not carried out.

Though concerning and dangerous behaviour on its own, it is important to know that excessive exercise may be an indication of the presence of a disorder.

- People with anorexia nervosa commonly engage in excessive exercise as a way to control their body weight and shape.
- People with bulimia nervosa sometimes engage in excessive exercise as a form of compensation following a binge eating episode.
- Excessive exercise can present as a symptom in other atypical eating disorders as a way to control weight/shape or as a compensatory behavior.
- If the exercise of choice primarily consists of lifting weights, or exercise that increases muscle mass, the person might also be experiencing muscle dysmorphia. (For more information, please see chapter 16: Bigorexia: Muscle Dysmorphia in Young People.)

PROBLEMATIC GYM CULTURE

In western countries, there is an increasingly problematic culture developing in certain gyms and social circles. This is exacerbated by social media outlets such as Instagram, Facebook and Tumblr. This problematic gym culture involves promoting 'fitspo' (fitness inspiration) slogans endorsing extreme and excessive exercising. Extreme exercise is very dangerous; partly due to this culture of pushing your body to its limits, or 'no pain, no gain' mentality, there has recently been a rise in the number of cases of severe muscle damage and even muscle 'melting' (a very serious condition called rhabdomyolysis, which can lead to kidney damage in some cases). Coupled with excessive dietary restrictions, there is severe cause for concern. The body is being pushed too hard and fast for it to repair properly, especially if the person's body has not been conditioned or trained over a period of time (as in the case of athletes) to cope with the increase in activity levels.

WARNING SIGNS/INDICATORS: WHEN 'HEALTHY' BEHAVIOURS BECOME 'UNHEALTHY'

In many cases it may be difficult to determine whether the young person is making healthy changes to their diet and/or exercise regimen for the purpose of improving their health, or whether they are displaying early warning signs for the development of dangerous and excessive dieting or exercising behaviours. It's made more difficult when these 'unhealthy' or 'excessive' changes are thought to be healthy changes to the individual. People who make extreme changes to their diet or their exercise routine usually tell their friends and family (and themselves) that they are doing it to improve their health. This section describes some warning signs to be mindful of to help you determine whether the changes that someone is making to their diet or exercise routine are potentially problematic.

Diet – signs to look out for:

- Reduction in food intake or skipping meals.
- Development of rules or rituals around eating and mealtimes, e.g. cutting up food into smaller pieces, only eating using particular tableware (i.e. specific plates, bowls or utensils), chewing for a specific number of times before swallowing, or consuming liquids in place of solids.
- Adoption of new dietary requirements, e.g. vegetarian, vegan, paleo, gluten-free, low/no carb, low/no sugar, low/no fat.
- Counting calories.
- Weighing food.
- Eating in secret.
- Obsession with 'healthy' eating.
- Division of food into 'good' and 'bad' food.
- Chewing and spitting (CHSP) out food that they see as 'forbidden' or 'bad'.
- Dieting to gain weight: although less common, another concerning diet involves overeating with the purpose of gaining weight or 'bulking up'. These types of diets can be high in fat, carbohydrates and proteins. This sort of problematic eating more commonly occurs in males attempting to gain muscle mass.

Aside from the more obvious symptoms related to the person's eating habits and weight changes, some other symptoms you might notice if someone is dieting are:

- Irritability.
- Hunger.
- Fatigue.
- Depressed mood.
- Increased interest and focus on food, meal planning and eating.

Exercise – signs to look out for:

- Continuing to exercise when feeling unwell, or when injured.
- Not allowing adequate time to rest and recover between workouts.
- Missing social functions to exercise.
- Firmly adhering to an obsessive exercise regimen.
- Anxious/distressed/upset if unable to exercise as planned.
- Ever-increasing intensity or duration.
- Exercising 'to make up for' consumed food.

Apart from the above, some other symptoms you might notice if someone is exercising an unhealthy amount are:

- Increased interest/obsession with exercise, and their physique.
- Withdrawal from social activity (prioritising their exercise regimen).
- Injury, strain, muscle pain or muscle fatigue.
- Physical agitation.
- Dehydration.
- Physical exhaustion and fatigue.

WHY DO THESE 'EXCESSIVE' BEHAVIOURS DEVELOP?

1. To make a change to physical appearance

The young person may have experienced criticism of their appearance from a peer, friend, member of their family or other person, or the young person may have perceived 'problems' in their appearance due to other influences such as the media, or by comparing themselves to their peers or to their role models (this doesn't have to be a 'celebrity': it can be a parent or guardian). The young person decides to take action to change their appearance by adjusting their diet or their exercise, but does so in a dangerous and unhealthy manner.

2. As a mechanism for control

Adolescence is a difficult time, full of many changes, and there can be a lot of pressure on young people to conform to a certain standard. It's common for young people to feel like their world is changing too rapidly or that things have got out of control. Some people find comfort in being able to control their eating and levels of activity when they are having difficulty controlling other aspects of their lives.

TREATMENT FOR EXCESSIVE DIETING AND EXERCISE

Treatment involves working with a professional (psychologist, dietitian and/or exercise physiologist) to get education on healthy versus unhealthy behaviours, to get support, and to create a plan to eliminate unhealthy rules, rituals and behaviours, and to commence a lifestyle involving healthy eating practices and a healthy amount of exercise.

What you can do if you are concerned about someone's eating habits or exercise regimen

- Talk to them about it. Tell them that you are concerned about them and explain why.
- Seek advice from a support line (e.g. Beat, school counsellor, psychologist, or family doctor).
- Ask the young person what you can do to support them.

Authors' biographies

Brooke, Phillip, Amy and Andreea are all affiliated with the University of Sydney.

Brooke Donnelly is a Senior Clinical Psychologist and Network Eating Disorder Coordinator at Royal Prince Alfred Hospital in Sydney. Phillip Aouad is a psychology PhD candidate whose research focuses on unexplored eating disorder symptoms. Amy Burton and Andreea Heriseanu are Clinical Psychology Interns and PhD candidates.

See also:

Chapter 6: Understanding Self-harm

Chapter 12: Understanding Eating Disorders in Young People

Recommended organisations and websites:

Eating Disorder Hope www.eatingdisorderhope.com/information/orthorexia-excessive-exercise

The British Dietetic Association: www.bda.uk.com

NHS: www.nhs.uk/Livewell/Goodfood

National Centre for Eating Disorders: eating-disorders.org.uk

Beat: www.beateatingdisorders.org.uk

    Helpline: Adult 0808 801 0677; Youthline 0808 801 0711

Men Get Eating Disorders Too: www.mengetedstoo.co.uk

The Mix: www.themix.org.uk/your-body/fitness-and-diet

For more online resources visit:
generationnext.com.au/handbook

14. ANOREXIA NERVOSA

**Brooke Donnelly, Phillip Aouad,
Amy Burton & Andreea Heriseanu**

This chapter will provide an overview of anorexia nervosa in adolescents, how to recognise it, and what to do for support. Anorexia nervosa is associated with a range of serious physical and emotional consequences, hence early intervention is critical in order to reach full recovery.

INTRODUCTION

Eating disorders are common mental illnesses. Anorexia nervosa ('anorexia') is a serious mental illness that affects approximately one in 200 girls and women over their lifetime, and approximately one in 2000 boys and men. Anorexia is characterised by extreme weight loss due to behaviours such as restriction of food intake, laxative use, excessive exercise or self-induced vomiting. An important feature of anorexia is the denial of the seriousness of the weight loss.

Young people are at the highest risk of developing an eating disorder during adolescence, a time of significant change. As this is a time of increased vulnerability, eating disorders can damage physical, emotional, social and neurological development and some young sufferers do not reach their full potential in these areas if they don't receive treatment quickly enough. However, anorexia can be confusing for parents, teachers, friends and loved ones to identify and understand; unlike a lot of other mental illnesses, the young person usually wants to avoid treatment and be left alone.

Anorexia is more than a severe mental illness. It carries the risk of significant medical complications, and psychological features of the disorder include: depression often as a result of starvation, irritability, obsessional thinking and behaviour, reduced concentration and social withdrawal.

In this chapter we will outline the symptoms and behaviours to look out for and how you can support a young person who might be suffering with this mental illness. We will also discuss the diagnostic features of anorexia, reiterate the importance of early intervention and describe evidence-based treatments.

WHAT IS ANOREXIA NERVOSA?

The term 'anorexia nervosa' was coined by Sir William Gull, a prominent English physician, in 1874. According to the DSM-5 (*Diagnostic and Statistical Manual* – fifth edition), which is the manual used by most clinicians and researchers to diagnose mental illnesses, the criteria for anorexia are:

1. **The ongoing restriction of energy intake leading to significantly low body weight, in relation to what is minimally expected for age, sex, developmental trajectory and physical health.**
   - The severity of anorexia in terms of weight loss is calculated using the expected body weight (EBW) and where the young person's weight sits in the percentile range for their age and sex.
   - EBW is different from the calculation used to determine an adult's body mass index (BMI).
   - EBW is the assumed or 'ideal' weight of a young person compared to their age- and sex-matched peers. A low-percentage EBW is considered to be less than 75 per cent of expected body weight. For example, if a young person is expected to weigh 50 kilograms and they weigh below 37.5 kilograms, then they are considered to have a low EBW.

- Many factors can come into effect when considering a significantly low body weight. For more information see: World Health Organization: Child Growth Standards (2006) – available from www.who.int/childgrowth/standards/en.

2. **Disturbance in the way one's body weight or shape is experienced, undue influence of body shape and weight on self-evaluation, or persistent lack of recognition of the seriousness of the current low body weight.**
   - While the young person may have a disturbed perception of their body image, they may not be able to recognise that they have an issue (showing poor insight and judgement).
   - Disturbed perception of body image may be expressed in a number of ways, such as:
     - Expressing concern over their body or weight.
     - Constantly weighing themselves.
     - Continuously checking their body in the mirror.
     - Inaccurately comparing their body to other individuals'.

There are two sub-types of anorexia nervosa:
- *Anorexia nervosa–restricting*: this is the most common type of anorexia, where the individual severely restricts their food intake. Restriction is highly variable; for example, it may involve maintaining a particular calorie count, restricting entire food groups, or eating only one meal a day. It often involves following obsessive and rigid rules, such as only eating foods of a particular colour, or 'safe' brands.
- *Anorexia nervosa binge-purge*: where the individual regularly engages in binge eating and/or purging behaviours.

In the early stages of anorexia it can be hard for parents, loved ones, friends or teachers to identify that there is a problem. The young person may persistently deny the presence of any weight or shape concern to hide or conceal the illness. It is important to highlight that while anorexia is a serious mental illness with significant medical consequences, for some young people the presence of the illness does not result in a detrimental effect on their academic or competitive sport performance; in fact, it can translate into an opposite effect. This is part of the insidious nature of the illness: to narrow the scope of the young person's attention to areas of their life where they feel more in control, harnessing perfectionism and obsessive behaviours.

For more information on risk factors for an eating disorder, please see chapter 12.

AREN'T SOME PEOPLE 'NATURALLY THIN'?

There are certainly some cultural groups that are genetically predisposed to having a body composition characterised by a higher ratio of lean muscle tissue to adipose tissue (fat), which means their basal metabolic rate is slightly higher. In other words, some cultural groups may be slightly more muscular and, therefore, their bodies are more efficient at using energy. However, for most of us the basic rule is that our body weight is a result of energy in, energy out. If a young person is underweight, and there is no medical reason that would explain ongoing or recent weight loss, the most likely explanation is the obvious one: they aren't taking in enough energy and/or they are exercising too much. Maintaining a low weight places anyone, especially an adolescent, at risk of a wide range of serious health consequences.

WHY ARE ADOLESCENTS AT RISK?

While overall incidence rates of anorexia have not increased over past decades, there has been an increase in the high-risk age group of fifteen- to nineteen-year-old females. It is unclear whether this reflects better screening, detection and diagnosis, or whether this is an actual increase in the number of young women developing anorexia.

Puberty is a high-risk time for adolescents with regards to a range of health issues. However, the changes occurring within one's body – both hormonally and in terms of physical appearance – are believed to precipitate an elevated period of risk for the onset of an eating disorder. The big picture is that puberty presents a time of immense change, which can be very difficult for some young people. If a young person has a predisposition to anxiety or a personality trait of perfectionism, this can be exacerbated during their teenage years. If a young person experiences distressing events, such as relationship break-ups or bullying, or perceives normal life events, such as academic performance, to be overly stressful, one way to feel more in control of their life can be through dieting or exercise. This, coupled with perfectionism or an anxiety disorder, can present a dangerous path to the onset of an eating disorder.

WHAT ARE SOME OF THE OTHER THINGS A YOUNG PERSON WITH ANOREXIA MIGHT BE STRUGGLING WITH?

- Low mood or depression.
- Anxiety, including obsessive-compulsive disorder.
- Social or relationship disturbances.
- Anhedonia: a loss of pleasure in things that the individual usually enjoyed pre-illness.
- Impaired set shifting, i.e. a concrete and rigid approach to shifting 'rules'.
- Reduced energy, decreased concentration and executive functioning (such as planning, focusing, juggling multiple tasks successfully).
- Self-harm or suicidal ideation.

Some of the features of the above problems and disorders can be explained by, or worsened, by the effects of starvation or malnutrition in anorexia.

WARNING SIGNS

The following is a list of some of the behaviours or physical changes that you might see in a young person who is experiencing anorexia, or is at risk of developing anorexia:

- **Increasingly focused on body shape and/or weight** – puberty can make anyone self-conscious; however, issues arise when the young person becomes fixated on, obsessed or markedly concerned about their body shape or weight.
- **Changes to eating and exercise** – be wary of major changes to eating and changes to exercise regimes. Dieting behaviour (e.g. monitoring energy intake on an app, following a fad diet, suddenly becoming vegan, avoiding food groups such as carbohydrates) should raise concern. Be curious about your child's language, e.g. if they are categorising foods as 'good' or 'bad' – what does this mean to them and has it changed their eating? Refer to chapter 13: 'Excessive Dieting and Exercise' for more information about this.
- **Developing rules and/or rituals around eating and meals** – these may include completing certain actions in a particular order, needing to do something a particular number of times, or having items of food not touching, or cutting food into bite-sized pieces.
- **Secret eating and/or exercise** – people with an eating disorder may only eat or exercise when alone, or may only eat certain foods in secret.
- **Preoccupation with food** – cooking, reading food blogs, watching cooking programmes.
- **Strange food-related behaviours** – a common example is hoarding food but not eating it or preparing elaborate cakes or meals for others without consuming any.
- **Physical agitation** – fidgeting and restlessness could be due to hunger or could be seen by the young person as a way to burn more energy.

- **Weight loss** – this isn't always easy to spot as it can be hidden by wearing baggy clothes or by layering of clothes.
- **Social media usage** – a lot of material online and on social media outlets can be a bad influence on people who are vulnerable to the development of eating disorders. There is serious cause for concern if the young person is accessing 'pro-ana' material ('pro-ana' refers to a subculture that praises and promotes anorexia), or if the person is looking at and/or posting 'fitspo' or 'thinspo' material (material which aims to 'inspire' thinness or fitness, usually images of people's bodies).
- **Compulsive or excessive exercising** – much like food intake, there can be a strict set of rigid rules around exercise that a young person might be adhering to. This can translate into exercising despite illness or injury; exercising despite extreme weather; experiencing distress if exercise is not possible.
- **Complaining of bloating**, constipation, or developing self-diagnosed food intolerances.
- **Repetitive or obsessive behaviours** relating to body shape and weight (e.g. repeated weighing, looking in the mirror obsessively and pinching waist or wrists).
- **Apparent low body temperature** – feeling cold most of the time, even on warm days; some young people will wear warm clothes inappropriate for weather.
- **Wearing loose clothes** to conceal weight loss – there may be overlap with the point above, i.e. some young people suffering from anorexia will experience low body temperature and 'rug up' even on warm days, while others will wear loose clothes or additional layers to conceal their appearance and/or weight loss.
- **Irritability**.
- **Fainting or dizziness**.
- **Fine hair appearing** on face and body (lanugo).
- **Social withdrawal** and relationship disturbances.

THE COST OF ANOREXIA

The burden of anorexia (and, indeed, any eating disorder) has impacts that go beyond just the individual. With over 920 000 Australians thought to have an eating disorder, the estimated total socioeconomic cost of eating disorder care, in 2012, was approximately seventy billion dollars. Moreover, although the NHS may provide psychiatric care, many families opt to pay or use private insurance to care for their loved one. Therefore, given the increased chance of relapse if treatment is delayed, it is also financially beneficial in the long run to get help as early as possible.

Quality of life (for individuals and loved ones)

Despite the fact that eating disorders can severely affect an individual's life, the impact of the disorder can unintentionally branch out and also affect those around a sufferer. Worry about a young person with an eating disorder can affect parents' and carers' own quality of life. Moreover, they may feel helpless or powerless to do anything to change the situation, and may feel guilty about not recognising the disease earlier, or feel responsible for the child developing the disorder in the first place. At this stage it is important to remember that the young person is having a hard time controlling the disordered thoughts. They may, in fact, feel incredibly guilty yet powerless themselves. A gentle and supportive approach needs to be taken when discussing concerns related to eating disorders.

Do not blame yourself or the child for the eating disorder or other associated issues (such as anxiety and depression). Know that there is help and support available for both the young person, and for the family. Start by looking at the resources in this book, followed by talking to your family doctor, school counsellor, or other mental health professional. They will be able to guide you towards the best approach and support your child in the best manner.

WHAT ARE THE PHYSICAL EFFECTS OF ANOREXIA?

Extreme dieting and weight loss can have serious and ongoing effects on any individual, especially in developing children and teens, for whom optimal nutrition is crucial.

Anorexia has an impact on virtually every single organ and body system. Some of the more common effects of poor nutrition on the development of young people may involve the:

- **Cardiovascular system:** feeling cold, low blood pressure causing dizziness/fainting, irregular heartbeat.
- **Hormonal system:** fatigue, weakened immune response, hair loss, low blood sugar, decreased thyroid function, metabolite imbalances.
- **Gastrointestinal system:** digestion difficulties (such as chronic constipation), acid reflux, irritable bowel syndrome, bloating.
- **Haematological (blood composition) system:** vitamin and mineral disturbances (such as anaemia).
- **Hair, nail and skin:** issues due to poor nutrition (such as lanugo – fine hairs that grow mainly on the arms, chest and face as a way for the body to preserve heat in the absence of body fat).
- **Muscular system:** loss of muscle mass.
- **Neurological/cognitive (brain) system:** movement difficulties, cognitive difficulties (such as loss of motivation, and loss of goal-directed behaviour), memory loss, 'brain fog', disorientation.
- **Renal (kidneys):** low potassium and sodium, and oedema (swelling, usually in the legs, due to the accumulation of fluid).
- **Reproductive system:** loss of menstruation in females, reduced sperm count in males.
- **Skeletal (including teeth):** tooth decay and gum damage, osteopenia and osteoporosis.

It is important to keep in mind that most of the symptoms mentioned above may be resolved with the restoration of the young person to a normal weight and good nutrition.

EARLY INTERVENTION IS CRITICAL FOR ANOREXIA

We can define early intervention as: *the taking of action towards a situation or issue before it has any further time to develop, worsen, or become irreversible.* Therefore, in terms of intervening early when it comes to anorexia, evidence-based treatment delivered by trained professionals needs to be taken as soon as possible, once the problem has been identified. Early intervention leads to a reduction of severity, duration of illness and the long-term impacts of the disorder. Moreover, it may help to reduce the rate of relapse later in life.

The first step in seeking treatment for anorexia is for the young person to complete a thorough medical assessment with a paediatrician or GP, in addition to a psychological assessment with a clinical psychologist (specialising in eating disorder treatment) or psychiatrist. This is because of the serious medical consequences that can occur from anorexia, the complex nature of this mental illness and the high rates of related problems that require specialist assessment to reach a clear diagnostic picture. For example, an assessment of the progression of symptoms up until the point of assessment, and an evaluation of the severity and frequency of the young person's symptoms, are critical pieces of information that will inform their treatment.

The treatment experience of a young person with anorexia is highly variable. This is partly due to the inherent ambivalence towards change and recovery from anorexia that is characteristic of this mental illness. It is also partly due to the huge range of available, evidence-based treatments depending on the geographical location (metropolitan areas vs regional and rural areas) of the young person. It is a sad fact that some young people will suffer from negative attitudes from health professionals due to the stigma associated with eating disorders.

WHAT CAN YOU DO IF YOU THINK SOMEONE YOU KNOW HAS ANOREXIA?

- Talk to them in an open, empathetic, non-judgemental way. Eating disorder symptoms are difficult to discuss, so it is essential to build trust.
- Alternatively, encourage them to talk to another trusted person.
- Help them to seek information/treatment (see resources at the end of this book).
- If they are suffering from any of the warning signs listed in this chapter, suggest they see a health professional immediately.
- Be aware of the way you talk about body image, how you approach food and eating in general.
- If you feel overwhelmed, seek professional, specialist help (see resources).

Anorexia is an insidious illness and unlike most other mental illness, it is *egosyntonic* (the thoughts and behaviours associated with the illness are in line with the person's values or ideal self-image). Therefore, it can be highly distressing for a young person suffering with anorexia to be presented with reasons why they need to change or have treatment.

The 'big picture' of treatment for anorexia is that early intervention is key, and a multidisciplinary approach is critical with clear, regular communication between all parties, including, of course, the young person and their family. Below is a listing of the latest evidence-based treatments for anorexia:

- Initially, weekly sessions with a medical practitioner such as a GP or paediatrician to monitor physical health, until there is no evidence of abnormal medical signs (such as low heart rate or low blood pressure) or medical tests (such as low electrolytes) which can occur when the condition is getting severe, at which time the frequency of medical appointments can decrease.

- **Family-Based Treatment (FBT) for anorexia:** this is the evidence-based 'gold standard' in terms of treatment for an adolescent with any eating disorder. It is an outpatient treatment where the family is the primary resource to re-nourish the young person or normalise their eating patterns. Critically, the young person should also receive therapy sessions once their eating and weight has normalised, to address normal adolescent concerns that may trigger a relapse if not addressed.
- **Cognitive Behaviour Therapy for Eating Disorders (CBT-E):** this treatment focuses on the factors that are maintaining the illness, not the factors that were responsible for its development. Regular eating and monitoring weight are key components.
- **Specialist eating disorder day programmes:** usually offering CBT-E, this is an intensive form of outpatient treatment where the young person receives between four to eight hours of group-based therapy from a Multidisciplinary Team (MDT) of clinical psychologists, dietitians, occupational therapists, social workers, nurses and psychiatrists between three to six days per week for a period of usually four to eight weeks. The intervention is designed to address the specific barriers adolescents with an eating disorder experience by increasing their capacity to cope with distress and the challenge of eating.
- **Specialist eating disorder inpatient programmes:** similar to the day programme description above, inpatient treatment programmes use an MDT approach to offer intensive nutritional refeeding, behavioural support and psychological treatment in either a public or private setting. Daily medical monitoring is at the centre of treatment and its necessity is often the reason for admission.
- **Pharmacological treatment:** in cases where the young person has significant depression or anxiety, medication may be used to address these symptoms. Depression and anxiety are known to complicate treatment response in anorexia.

- **E-therapy:** this is an emerging treatment modality with good acceptability for adolescents, due to their familiarity with technology, usually in the form of CBT adapted for internet delivery, or CBT in a non-specialist guided self-help form. A degree of anonymity, convenience and accessibility go hand in hand with e-therapies. In regional and rural areas where a local eating disorder specialist clinician or team isn't available, this form of treatment is an effective option, delivered in conjunction with regular physician or GP appointments.

TAKE-HOME MESSAGES FOR PARENTS

- If you are unsure whether to be concerned or seek professional help, err on the side of caution. A good place to start is with your family physician or GP, seeing them with your child, to discuss your concerns transparently and respectfully.
- Severe weight loss associated with dietary restriction can be life-threatening.
- It is critical to seek treatment as soon as possible. The research is clear: the earlier treatment is started, the better the outcomes will be for your child.
- Externalise the illness: label the anorexia as 'the anorexia'. The illness is *not* your child and your child is not the illness. Young people who have recovered from anorexia have reported that having their loved ones separate them from the anorexia supports them in untangling which are *their* thoughts and wishes, versus the thoughts and wishes of the anorexia. At the early stages of the illness your child may rail against this; however, this reflects the egosyntonic nature of anorexia.
- You are not to blame for the illness. However, you *do* have a central role to play in seeking the best treatment possible for your child.

- It is okay to seek a second opinion if you are concerned about your child's health. You are their parent and have their best interests at heart. If your parental intuition tells you that the current treatment plan is not satisfactory or a good 'fit' for your child and your family, discuss your concerns with the treating team. There may be ways that the existing treatment can be adapted that will help achieve better outcomes for everyone involved.

- Your role is critical in helping your child overcome a major, life-threatening mental illness. Therefore, you may benefit from seeking your own support, for example, seeing an individual psychologist to bolster you in your ongoing role as a firm, empathetic and loving parent.

- Be aware of your own eating and exercise habits. Don't engage in any dieting, weight or 'fat' talk with your child. Model normal, flexible eating, i.e. three meals and two to three snacks per day plus appropriate fluid intake. Don't get caught up in food fads and try not to label foods as 'good', 'bad' or 'healthy'. *Food is food*. Eat widely from a range of different food groups and types.

- It can be challenging to be in the spotlight with regards to your own eating; if you need additional support around this, see an eating disorders specialist psychologist for guidance.

- Beat is the UK's leading charity supporting those affected by eating disorders and campaigning on their behalf. Its comprehensive website (www.beateatingdisorders.org.uk) contains advice for parents and carers supporting someone with an eating disorder.

TAKE-HOME MESSAGES FOR TEACHERS AND SCHOOL COUNSELLORS/YOUTH WORKERS

- A National Eating Disorder Collaboration report in Australia advises that approximately half of adolescent girls have tried to lose weight and practise extreme weight loss behaviours such as fasting, self-induced vomiting and smoking.

- As many as 75 per cent of high school girls 'feel fat' or want to lose weight.
- Young people who diet are six times more likely to develop an eating disorder; those who are severe dieters are eighteen times more likely to develop an eating disorder.
- Self-education and knowledge is critical. If you are better informed, you will be increasingly mindful and armed with skills to identify behaviours and risk factors in the young people you work with.
- Don't engage in any dieting, weight or 'fat' talk with young people. Model normal eating if you are eating with them.
- Beat offers training and CPD events for Schools, workplaces and primary care facilities in the UK. For more information, see www.beateatingdisorders.org.uk/training-cpd.

Author biography

Brooke, Phillip, Amy and Andreea are all affiliated with the University of Sydney.

Brooke Donnelly is a Senior Clinical Psychologist and Network Eating Disorder Coordinator at Royal Prince Alfred Hospital in Sydney. Phillip Aouad is a psychology PhD candidate whose research focuses on unexplored eating disorder symptoms. Amy Burton and Andreea Heriseanu are Clinical Psychology Interns and PhD candidates.

See also:

Chapter 5: Depression in Young People
Chapter 6: Understanding Self-harm
Chapter 7: Suicide and Attempted Suicide
Chapter 12: Understanding Eating Disorders in Young People
Chapter 13: Excessive Dieting and Exercise
Chapter 15: Bulimia and Binge Eating
Chapter 16: Bigorexia: Muscle Dysmorphia in Young People
Chapter 17: Fostering a Positive Body Image

Recommended organisations and websites:

National Centre for Eating Disorders: eating-disorders.org.uk

NHS: nhs.uk/Conditions/Anorexia

Anorexia and Bulimia care: www.anorexiabulimiacare.org.uk

Beat: www.beateatingdisorders.org.uk

    Helpline: 0808 801 0677; Youthline 0808 801 0711 (free)

Men Get Eating Disorders Too: www.mengetedstoo.co.uk

Further reading:

Grilo, C & Mitchell, JE 2010, *The Treatment of Eating Disorders: A Clinical Handbook*, The Guildford Press, New York.

Waller, G et al 2007, *Cognitive Behavioural Therapy for Eating Disorders*, Cambridge University Press (Medicine), Cambridge.

For more online resources visit:
generationnext.com.au/handbook

15. BULIMIA AND BINGE EATING

**Andreea Heriseanu, Brooke Donnelly,
Amy Burton & Phillip Aouad**

This chapter will provide an overview of bulimia nervosa and other binge eating disorders in adolescents, signs to help recognise these disorders, and what to do for support. While bulimia and binge eating can be severe and affect a young person's life, complete recovery is possible.

INTRODUCTION

Eating disorders are serious mental illnesses. They are a leading cause of burden of disease both in Australia and worldwide, and carry the highest mortality rate of any mental illness. They affect females and males of all shapes and sizes, and occur across all races and ethnic groups. Bulimia nervosa ('bulimia') is an eating disorder characterised by food binges, combined with compensatory behaviour such as purging, with a high personal value placed on shape and weight. Bulimia nervosa affects about one to two in 100 girls, and around one in 200 boys. Additionally, it is estimated that about 30 per cent of Australians aged between fifteen to twenty-four engage in food binges, and that about 14 per cent engage in purging behaviour.

Adolescence is a time of increased risk for developing problematic eating patterns, due to it being a time of rapid change. Physically, the body grows and develops towards adulthood; brain maturation is in process; socially, young people start to attend more to peers; norms and peer pressure for how to look and act become more pronounced. This is also the time when many young people start romantic and sexual relationships. Overall, body image starts to matter much more, and the perceived necessity to conform to societal physical standards increases. This, in turn, can lead to the development of bulimia, binge eating disorder and other eating difficulties.

Bulimia and binge eating affect more than a young person's eating, shape and weight. They can have a serious impact on overall physical and mental health, and on social and educational development. A high level of comorbidity (the presence of more than one disorder or issue of concern) is very common, with young people being at higher risk of suicide, and frequently experiencing depression, anxiety and substance use issues alongside their eating disorder.

Although bulimia and binge eating can be severe and have a widespread impact, support and effective treatments are available. As with most mental illnesses, early intervention is critical. Therefore, it is important for parents, teachers, and others who work with young people to learn to recognise the warning signs and symptoms, and know where to get help.

WHAT ARE BULIMIA, BINGE EATING DISORDER AND BINGE EPISODES?

Bulimia nervosa is a mental illness characterised by repeated episodes of binge eating associated with a sense of loss of control, which are combined with the use of compensatory behaviours. These are behaviours that the young person does in an effort to counteract the effects of the binge, such as fasting, vomiting, laxative abuse, diuretic usage and excessive exercise. Bulimia also involves placing high value on one's weight and shape for self-evaluation, which in turn maintains this illness. Medical complications of bulimia include: dehydration, severe tooth decay, digestive issues and heart problems. Binge eating disorder (BED) is a mental illness which is similar to bulimia, except individuals do not vomit or engage in any compensatory behaviours after they binge, which places them at higher risk of becoming overweight or obese.

Binge episodes are the hallmark feature of bulimia and BED. There are two types of binges: *objective* binge episodes and *subjective* binge episodes. People usually binge in secret due to the feelings of distress, guilt and shame associated with eating. According to the *Diagnostic and Statistical Manual of Mental Disorders* (DSM-5), an episode of objective binge eating is characterised by both:

1. Eating, in a discrete period of time (e.g. within any two-hour period), an amount of food that is **definitely larger** than most people would eat during a **similar period of time** and under **similar circumstances**, and;
2. A sense of **loss of control** over one's eating during the episode (e.g. a feeling that they cannot stop eating, even though they want to).

An *objective* binge episode (OBE) is where the amount of food consumed is definitely and objectively larger than what a similar person could consume in similar circumstances, and it occurs in a discrete period of time, rather than grazing on amounts of food over the course of the day. If you're unsure whether binges fall in this category, consider whether the amount of food eaten, when compiled on a table, would look reasonable for an average person to consume in one sitting. If not, it's probably an OBE.

Conversely, a *subjective* binge episode (SBE) is where the amount of food eaten is much less than that described in an OBE. It may consist of a chocolate bar or two sweet biscuits, perhaps more; however, in the context of a highly restrictive diet, this can represent an extremely distressing loss of control.

Loss of control over eating is an important eating disorder symptom which is linked with more comorbidity and decreased mental and social functioning – regardless of the amount of food eaten. It reflects a feeling that a person can't stop eating once they've started, or can't prevent themselves from eating in the first place. This experience can be very distressing to a young person.

Although it might be initially hard to tell the difference between a SBE and 'normal' overeating, the critical feature to consider is whether a sense of a loss of control is present and how that affected the young person's mood.

It's important to note that binges look very different from the normal points in time when we can all overeat, such as at special family celebrations or as part of religious celebrations such as Christmas, Sukkot, Diwali or the end of Ramadan, Eid al-Fitr. Research on the experience of binge eating is clear: the sense of a loss of control over one's eating is the primary difference between normative overeating and binge episodes, and leads to low mood and feelings of shame, guilt and disgust. The actual amount of food is less important.

DESCRIPTIONS OF BINGE EPISODES

- 'I continued to eat even though I was no longer hungry, and ate until I was uncomfortably full.'
- 'I thought I'd "blown it", so I might as well keep eating.'
- 'While eating, I felt I was in my own little world, or in a trance, and I couldn't do anything other than eat.'
- 'I felt helpless about controlling my eating.'
- 'I felt a sense of release while I was eating, but felt ashamed and disgusted afterwards.'

With bulimia, episodes of binge eating are coupled with the use of compensatory behaviours. These are actions taken by the young person intended to cancel, or 'undo' the effects of binge eating. Common compensatory behaviours include inducing vomiting following a binge episode, and fasting, or restricting how much food is eaten between binge episodes (the young person may also be involved in restrictive 'fad' diets). Other common compensatory behaviours include laxative abuse (intended to increase bowel movement), diuretic ('water pill') usage (for decreasing weight by eliminating water from the body), inappropriate use of other medication (prescription or over-the-counter) to control weight, and excessive, compulsive or 'driven' exercise (see chapter 13: 'Excessive Dieting and Exercise'). Compensatory behaviours are not effective for weight loss. In fact, they can contribute to weight gain over time, and can be both mentally and physically harmful.

PREVALENCE OF BULIMIA AND BINGE EATING

- In total, it is estimated that 29.3 per cent of Australians aged between fifteen and twenty-four years old engage in objective binge episodes on a regular basis.
- It is estimated that 1–2 per cent of young females are suffering from bulimia; less is known about the rates of bulimia in young men. Australian estimates suggest that 13.6 per cent of fifteen to twenty-four year olds engage in purging behaviour.
- It is estimated that 2–3 per cent of Australians suffer from BED, with 30–50 per cent of cases of BED being male. Compared to anorexia and bulimia, BED is not often thought of as a condition that affects teens as it typically develops in early adulthood; however, it can also begin earlier (or later) in life for some people.
- Prevalence of BED in Australia has doubled in the past decade.
- It is estimated that 1.9 per cent of Australians would meet criteria for an atypical eating disorder.

Source: *APA, 2013; Hay et al., 2008*

WHAT CAUSES BULIMIA AND BINGE EATING?

As with all mental health difficulties, there is not one single factor that causes bulimia, binge eating or any other type of eating disorder. The cause is a complex combination of personal or genetic vulnerabilities, exposure to risk factors, and/or lack of protective factors and helpful coping strategies. However, there are some known factors that place a young person at increased risk of developing bulimia or another binge-related problem.

Physical factors include:

- The onset of puberty, with the associated hormonal, body and brain changes.
- Heredity: a family history of eating disorders.
- Sex: although eating disorders including bulimia are on the rise in males, they are still much more common in females.

Psychological factors include:

- Low self-esteem.
- Placing high value on high achievement and on others' opinions.
- Perfectionism.
- Competitiveness.
- Impulsivity.
- Avoidance or fear of conflict.
- Difficulty expressing emotions such as anger, sadness, anxiety or fear.
- A lack of helpful coping strategies for difficult feelings.

There are also external factors that can contribute to the risk of developing bulimia and binge eating:

- Dieting is one of the main risk factors for developing any eating disorder. Recurrent dieting usually leads to weight gain or 'yo-yo' weight fluctuations.
- Life events, especially stressful events involving major life changes (e.g. loss of a loved one, parental separation, moving house or changing schools) can serve to trigger eating disorders.
- Sexual, physical or emotional abuse.

- Sociocultural factors such as attitudes towards body appearance and 'ideal looks' can also augment risk – e.g. prevailing western cultural values maintain the 'thin ideal' for women of all ages.
- Implicit messages about the high positive value of thinness and the importance of being a particular shape for males and females are constantly communicated through various types of media and advertising.

THE VICIOUS CYCLE OF BINGE EATING

It is believed that when a person has low self-esteem, and they highly value their weight or body shape (consistent with the thin/fit/muscular cultural ideal) they may use dieting in order to lose weight. In turn, dieting will lead to a 'starvation state' and cravings, which prompt binge eating. Bingeing will, however, increase the young person's concerns about shape and weight, and make them renew their dieting efforts, leading to a vicious cycle of restricting and bingeing. To counteract the effects of bingeing, the young person may turn to compensatory behaviours such as vomiting, which, together with bingeing, will further decrease self-esteem and increase attention placed on weight and shape, leading a vicious binge–purge cycle. Young people are especially vulnerable to this cycle during periods of low mood or depression, during times of interpersonal or relationship stress (e.g. following a relationship break-up), or when other negative or stressful events take place in their life.

CULTURAL MESSAGES AIMED AT MALES

The prevalence of eating disorders in males is on the rise. More than a quarter of males aged between eleven and twenty-four are dissatisfied with their appearance, and around two-thirds of twelve- to seventeen-year-old males report being involved in dieting to change their appearance.

Specific cultural messages aimed at this group represent an additional risk factor:

- 'Males should only have one body type: lean and muscular.' This unrealistic body ideal can lead to dieting and excessive exercise as boys and men attempt to conform.
- 'Males need to "take charge" and be in control.' When coping with difficult issues beyond their control, males can sometimes displace these anxieties onto their bodies, manifesting in control over the body through excessive exercise and dieting.
- 'Eating disorders and other mental illnesses are "weak", and not "masculine".' This type of message creates stigma around mental illness and interferes with treatment-seeking.

Generally, males who have bulimia will experience physical, psychological and social/educational difficulties similar to those of females with this illness. Therefore, the information contained within this chapter, including treatment options, is applicable to all bulimia sufferers regardless of gender.

HOW TO RECOGNISE BULIMIA AND BINGE EATING

Some common warning signs for bulimia are as follows:

Psychological signs
- Dissatisfaction with one's body, weight, shape or the look or size of particular body parts (e.g. stomach, hips).
- Distorted body image, e.g. a young person firmly believing they need to lose weight despite being a normal, healthy weight or even underweight; or the belief that a certain body part of area of the body is abnormal relative to the rest of their body, such as the thighs.

- Placing disproportionate value on physical appearance in terms of self-evaluation (e.g. 'I feel good about myself today because I look thin').
- Irritability or mood swings.

Behavioural signs

- Frequent visits to the toilet soon after meals.
- Frequent weighing or scrutinising of self in the mirror, or measuring oneself (taking a waist measurement, repeatedly trying on clothes, pinching oneself to determine amount of fat, etc).
- Choosing to eat alone, or refusing to eat meals with family or friends.
- Dieting behaviour (e.g. counting calories, avoiding entire food groups such as fats or carbohydrates, following a 'fad' diet, sudden and extreme changes to diet, such as becoming vegan).
- Excessive exercise (i.e. rigid regime, or exercising even when injured or unwell).
- Social withdrawal and problems with relationships.

Physical signs

- Substantial changes in weight that are not simply caused by growth spurts.
- 'Russell's Sign' (calluses or scarring on the knuckles or the back of the hand) can be present in people who repeatedly make themselves vomit.
- Fatigue or lethargy.
- Stomach pain, feeling bloated, and constipation.
- Oedema (swelling) can be present in people who use laxatives or diuretics.
- Irregular menstruation.
- Dental and mouth problems (such as wearing away of the enamel, or enlarged salivary glands) because of vomiting.
- Dizziness or fainting.
- Problems with sleep.

THE CONSEQUENCES OF BULIMIA AND BINGE EATING

Bulimia and binge eating are associated with lower quality of life, social impairment (isolation, withdrawal), poorer education and work functioning (missed days, decreased performance), and they also have a great impact on the person's overall health.

People who engage in binge eating and compensatory behaviours are at a higher risk of developing other significant mental and physical health problems compared to people who do not. Examples of conditions associated with bulimia and binge eating include:

- Other mental disorders, most commonly depressive disorders, anxiety disorders and substance abuse – this is explored in more detail below.
- Higher body mass index (BMI) and obesity.
- Chronic physical health conditions such as chronic pain, hypertension, diabetes and other metabolic complications.
- Cognitive (thinking) difficulties, impairment in concentration, 'brain fog'.
- Repeated purging impacts on physical health, contributing to issues such as: tooth decay, swollen face, acid reflux, digestive problems such as constipation, dehydration and potentially dangerous metabolite imbalances.

As a result, bulimia and binge eating have a high cost on the individual, family or carers, and society, due to expenses related to the treatment of the disordered eating itself, as well as associated health problems and loss in productivity.

Psychological comorbidity in bulimia and binge eating

A striking aspect of bulimia and BED is the high rate of co-occurring psychological disorders:

- Most prominent is depression, which is believed to occur in approximately 50 to 70 per cent of people with bulimia and

BED. Depressive symptoms (such as low self-esteem, self-loathing, shame or guilt) are common.

- Suicide risk is higher in those with bulimia than in the general population.
- Anxiety symptoms (e.g. fear of social situations) and anxiety disorders, such as obsessive-compulsive disorder (OCD), also co-occur.
- Bipolar spectrum disorders are often comorbid with bulimia.
- Alcohol and drug use is frequent (stimulant use is often an early attempt to control appetite and weight; binge episodes can also incorporate binge drinking, or alcohol may be used to cope with painful feelings).
- Features of emerging personality disorders can be present (such as borderline personality disorder, where there is difficulty managing emotions and impulses, relating to people and maintaining a stable self-image).

SUICIDE RISK

Signs to look out for:

- Feeling hopeless about the future.
- Feelings of isolation, loneliness and that no one cares.
- Using alcohol, drugs or non-prescribed medications.
- Self-harming behaviour, e.g. cutting, burning, hitting or constantly trying to put themselves in harm's way.
- Preparing for death by giving away possessions, writing goodbye letters, and setting affairs in order.
- Look out for these signs especially at times of loss, e.g. a break-up, a death in the family, etc.

Note: a young person is an increased risk of suicide when a friend or family member has recently committed suicide.

What to do:

- Take suicidal thoughts and intentions seriously.
- Remove obvious means (such as medication, alcohol, sharp knives, firearms if present).

- Do not avoid talking about suicide with the young person. It is a myth that asking about suicidal thoughts or behaviours will 'give them ideas'.
- Seek help from a trained professional such as a GP or a mental health professional.
- Call your local suicide hotline, Samaritans or Childline.
- For immediate help, go to the Accident and Emergency Department at your local hospital, contact your local child and adolescent mental health service or after-hours crisis team, or dial 999 or 112.
- See the 'Where to get help' section on page 198.

In summary, binge eating and bulimia (and associated problems) are serious conditions that adversely affect young people, often at a vulnerable point in their lives. Fortunately, effective evidence-based treatments are available for eating disorders; furthermore, low mood and anxiety symptoms are often resolved following effective treatment of the bulimia nervosa/binge eating itself.

WHAT TREATMENTS ARE AVAILABLE?

If a young person or their carer is concerned about eating, shape or weight issues, it is important to seek help from a trained professional as soon as possible, even if it is believed that the problem is only mild. A thorough assessment by a GP or paediatrician and a clinical psychologist or psychiatrist specialising in eating disorders is recommended. This specialist approach is important due to the complex nature of eating disorders and their serious potential medical complications, in addition to high levels of comorbidity, which can complicate diagnosis and treatment.

Several evidence-based treatments exist for binge eating and bulimia nervosa. It is recommended that these be used in conjunction with monitoring of the young person's physical health by a medical practitioner (through weighing, blood tests and heart function tests, etc.). For more detail about these treatments, please see the previous chapter:

- Family-based treatment (FBT)
- Cognitive Behaviour Therapy for eating disorders (CBT-E)
- Eating disorder day programmes
- Eating disorder inpatient programmes
- Pharmacological treatment
- E-therapy

CAN BULIMIA AND BINGE EATING BE PREVENTED?

While there is no known way to prevent binge eating and bulimia, early intervention is the best way to prevent the disorder from progressing. Knowing the signs of bulimia and disordered eating and seeking support can help prevent long-term health problems.

School programmes (such as 'Happy Being Me', by Dunstan, Paxton & McLean, 2016) have been developed for body dissatisfaction prevention within a school setting. These programmes address issues such as peer environments, media pressure to conform to physical ideals, social media, internalisation of appearance ideals, and body comparison. Such programs can help address some of the important contributors to the risk of developing an eating disorder.

Encouraging the use of helpful coping strategies by the young person can also be useful for mental health in general. These coping skills may include talking to trusted adults, self-care and relaxation, keeping a journal, hobbies, spending time with friends and assertiveness training.

TAKE-HOME MESSAGES FOR PARENTS

- Do not blame yourself.
- Talk to your child in a non-judgemental, open and accepting way.
- Encourage the young person to express their feelings and promote open communication at home, even if at times this can feel difficult.

- Check in with your child regularly, in a non-intrusive way.
- Help the young person to seek information/treatment (see 'Where to get help' section on page 198).
- Reassure the young person that gaining weight and changing body shape throughout adolescence are normal and healthy.
- Young people learn by example – try not to diet or skip meals, and model acceptance of different body types (including your own).
- Avoid labelling foods as 'good' or 'bad' as young people may feel guilty or ashamed if eating food designated as 'bad'.
- Avoid promoting unrealistic or overly perfectionistic goals in terms of grades and achievements, and reward effort instead.
- Encourage young persons to measure their value in terms of diverse personal attributes, and not physical appearance.
- Avoid using food as a reward, a bribe or a punishment.
- Allow the young person to eat when they are hungry and stop when they are full.
- If your child is not at medical risk, and they are undergoing regular physical check-ups by a GP or physician, gentle exercise such as walking, tai chi or some forms of yoga can be beneficial when social rather than solitary.
- Encourage physical exercise for enjoyment rather than for any perceived effects on weight and body shape.
- Discuss with young people the messages received through TV and other media and through social media (Instagram, Facebook, etc.), and help them build a critical awareness around these messages.
- Contact an online support group aimed at parents/carers of a child with an eating disorder (e.g. as offered by Beat: www.beateatingdisorder.org.uk/support-services/online-groups).
- If you continue to have concerns, or feel unable to reach out to your child, seek help from a qualified professional.
- Eating disorders affect more than just the young person. If you feel overwhelmed, it is important to get help yourself.

TAKE-HOME MESSAGES FOR TEACHERS AND SCHOOL COUNSELLORS/YOUTH WORKERS

- Contribute to a body-positive and inclusive school culture.
- Implement programmes aimed at increasing eating disorder literacy and at addressing body image concerns in the school environment.
- Provide an empathetic, supportive, non-judgemental space where young people can talk about their behaviours, thoughts and feelings.
- Talk to the young person in a non-judgemental way. Convey an open and accepting attitude to build trust.
- Encourage the young person to also talk to other trusted persons.
- Check in regularly, in a non-intrusive way.
- Help them to seek information/treatment.
- Be careful when discussing body image, food and dieting – young people use important adults such as teachers as role models.
- Obtain further training (such as through Beat). This is especially important for learning when to get other services/ professionals involved.

TAKE-HOME MESSAGES FOR HEALTH PROFESSIONALS

- The research is clear: if a young person has a positive treatment experience when they initially disclose symptoms of an eating disorder to a health professional, their treatment trajectory and rates of recovery at a five-year follow-up will be significantly better than those who have a negative treatment experience, e.g. if they perceive being judged or have their symptoms dismissed.

- If you're unsure whether you can help an adolescent with an eating disorder, be transparent about any real limitations of what you can do in your role.
- Through providing an encouraging, professional space for the young person to speak about their concerns in, and collaborating with other health professionals involved in the care of the young person, you will offer an invaluable positive treatment experience.
- This increases the likelihood of the young person seeking treatment again in the future for *any* mental health or general health condition.

Authors' biographies

Brooke, Phillip, Amy and Andreea are all affiliated with the University of Sydney.

Brooke Donnelly is a Senior Clinical Psychologist and Network Eating Disorder Coordinator at Royal Prince Alfred Hospital in Sydney. Phillip Aouad is a psychology PhD candidate whose research focuses on unexplored eating disorder symptoms. Amy Burton and Andreea Heriseanu are Clinical Psychology Interns and PhD candidates.

See also:

Chapter 4: Anxiety in Young People
Chapter 5: Depression in Young People
Chapter 6: Understanding Self-harm
Chapter 7: Suicide and Attempted Suicide
Chapter 12: Understanding Eating Disorders in Young People
Chapter 13: Excessive Dieting and Exercise
Chapter 14: Anorexia Nervosa
Chapter 16: Bigorexia: Muscle Dysmorphia in Young People
Chapter 17: Fostering a Positive Body Image

Recommended organisations and websites:

National Centre for Eating Disorders: eatingdisorders.org.uk
NHS: www.nhs.uk/conditions/Bulimia
Anorexia and Bulimia Care: www.anorexiabulimiacare.org.uk
Beat: www.beatingeatingdisorders.org.uk
   Helpline: 0808 801 0677; Youthline 0808 801 0711 (free)

Maudsley Parents: a US-based information and support website for parents of children with eating disorders www.maudsleyparents.org

Further reading:

American Psychiatric Association 2013, *Diagnostic and Statistical Manual of Mental Disorders: DSM-5*, American Psychiatric Publishing, Washington, DC.

Astrachan-Fletcher, E & Maslar, M 2009, *The Dialectical Behavior Therapy Skills Workbook for Bulimia*, New Harbinger Publications.

Fairburn, CG 2013, *Overcoming Binge Eating*, 2nd ed. Guildford Press, New York.

Hay, PJ, Mond, J, Buttner, P & Darby, A 2008, 'Eating Disorder Behaviors Are Increasing: Findings from Two Sequential Community Surveys in South Australia', *PLoS ONE*, vol. 3, no. 2, p 1541.

 For more online resources visit:
generationnext.com.au/handbook

16. BIGOREXIA: MUSCLE DYSMORPHIA IN YOUNG PEOPLE

Dr Scott Griffiths

This chapter provides an overview of muscle dysmorphia in adolescence. Readers will gain an understanding of what muscle dysmorphia is, how to recognise it, and what to do for support.

INTRODUCTION

Muscle dysmorphia is a mental disorder with many colourful monikers, including 'bigorexia', 'megarexia', 'musclerexia', and 'manorexia'. The simplest way to begin to understand muscle dysmorphia is to think of it as 'reverse anorexia'. In 'regular' anorexia, or anorexia nervosa, individuals are propelled towards thinness at any cost, and are frequently very thin with very low body weights. In muscle dysmorphia, individuals are propelled towards muscularity at any cost, and are frequently very muscular with very high body weights.

The distinction of muscularity versus thinness gives rise to several points of difference and similarity between muscle dysmorphia and anorexia. For example, in anorexia, the drugs that an individual may take in order to induce weight loss will typically include diuretics and laxatives, whereas in muscle dysmorphia, the drugs that are taken to induce muscle gain will typically include anabolic steroids and thermogenic drugs. Exercise provides another parallel. Individuals with muscle dysmorphia are more likely to lift weights (resistance training) while individuals with anorexia are more likely to run on a treadmill (cardiovascular training). Common to both anorexia and muscle dysmorphia, however, is that individuals with these disorders frequently use drugs in order to achieve their desired body. Similarly, individuals with these disorders frequently become compulsive exercisers, meaning that the exercise is used not only to burn calories or build muscle, but to regulate how one feels, including as a salve for anxiety and other negative emotions.

At this point, the reader might have surmised that there are gender differences in anorexia and muscle dysmorphia – and you would be correct. The few studies of muscle dysmorphia suggest that sufferers are mostly men and boys, and the more numerous studies of anorexia suggest that sufferers are mostly women and girls. The gender imbalance for each disorder reflects the different body types that are considered desirable for the different genders. For boys, the most desirable body is a muscular, V-shaped torso comprised of broad shoulders, a large chest, and a narrow waist. Boys additionally desire muscular arms, with particular attention paid to having big biceps, and desire a 'six-pack' of clearly visible abdominal muscles. Height may also factor into the equation – boys prefer to be tall over short. For girls, the most desirable body is much less muscular and is commonly described as 'thin' or 'skinny'. Although some girls may refer to their ideal body as 'toned', research suggests that there is a substantial difference in what boys and girls consider to be 'toned'. In general, girls desire an amount of muscle that is a great deal less than that preferred by most boys, who commonly describe their ideal body as 'ripped' or 'built', or even 'jacked'. This difference in body preferences is the main reason why most individuals with muscle dysmorphia are boys. It is important to recognise, however, that a considerable minority of individuals with anorexia are men (estimates range from 10 to 33 per cent), and it is likely that a considerable minority of individuals with muscle dysmorphia are women. The absence of information on women with muscle dysmorphia likely reflects the fact that the necessary research has not been conducted yet, not that girls with muscle dysmorphia do not exist.

We do not know how many people suffer from muscle dysmorphia because the type of evidence that is required for this knowledge – epidemiological evidence – has not been conducted. What we are certain of is that the number of individuals with muscle dysmorphia is likely increasing. The evidence in support of this comes from studies of anabolic steroids. Anabolic steroids are synthetic forms of the male sex hormone testosterone and they are singularly effective at building muscle – a property that makes them highly attractive to individuals with muscle dysmorphia. Since 2010, anabolic steroids have been the number one most commonly injected drug among *new* injection drug users, ahead of heroin, methamphetamine, opioids and cocaine. Nationwide, the proportion of injection drug users who reported that the last drug they injected was steroids increased from 2 per cent in 2010 to 7 per cent in 2015. The increase in the prevalence of steroid use in Australia likely parallels an increase in the prevalence of muscle dysmorphia because 40 to 50 per cent of individuals with muscle dysmorphia also use steroids.[1]

Understandably, the parents of adolescents and adolescents themselves may worry over the line at which thoughts and behaviours about muscularity cross over from 'okay' to 'not okay'. Researchers of muscle dysmorphia worry about these lines too – it accomplishes little if we unnecessarily pathologise otherwise normal thoughts and behaviours. It is normal that adolescents think about their bodies and may desire to change them. It is normal that adolescents may be enthusiastic about trying out weightlifting, especially if they have friends who also go to the gym. It has even been suggested that, for some adolescents, steroid use exists in the context of a general 'drug exploration', in which an adolescent tries many different illicit drugs, implying that steroid use is not necessarily linked to muscle dysmorphia or body image problems. Because muscle dysmorphia is a new mental disorder with little available research, it is challenging – and worrying – for parents and adolescents, particularly with regard to whether or not it is 'worth saying something'. In order to provide some clarity, the next section focuses on what muscle dysmorphia 'looks like', and attempts to distinguish muscle dysmorphia from non-clinical, non-problematic, otherwise benign adolescent interest in their appearance, diet and exercise.

WHAT IS MUSCLE DYSMORPHIA?

The diagnostic criteria for muscle dysmorphia proposed by Harrison Pope, the original 'discoverer' of the condition, are:

A. Preoccupation with the idea that one's body is not sufficiently lean and muscular. Characteristic associated behaviours include long hours of lifting weights and excessive attention to diet.

B. The preoccupation is manifested by at least two of the following four criteria:
   i. The individual frequently gives up important social, occupational, or recreational activities because of a compulsive need to maintain his or her workout and diet schedule.
   ii. The individual avoids situations in which his or her body is exposed to others, or endures such situations only with marked distress or intense anxiety.
   iii. The preoccupation about the inadequacy of body size or musculature causes clinically significant distress or impairment in social, occupational or other important areas of functioning.
   iv. The individual continues to work out, diet or use ergogenic (performance-enhancing) substances despite knowledge of adverse physical or psychological consequences.

C. The primary focus of the preoccupation and behaviours is on being too small or inadequately muscular, as distinguished from fear of being fat, as in anorexia nervosa, or a primary preoccupation only with other aspects of appearance as in other forms of body dysmorphic disorder.

Terms like 'preoccupation' are highly subjective and prone to misinterpretation – a subjectivity made all the more important because Criterion A, which states 'preoccupation with the idea that one's body is sufficiently lean and muscular', is arguably the defining feature of muscle dysmorphia. Preoccupation means that, for an individual with muscle dysmorphia, a considerable portion of each day is spent on thoughts or behaviours focused around the pursuit of a more muscular body. In studies, the average length of time that individuals with muscle dysmorphia spend thinking about getting bigger, being too small, or not being big enough, has ranged from 240 to 330 minutes each day – that equates to between four and five and a half hours each day. In comparison, individuals who go to the gym but do not have muscle dysmorphia spend just twenty to forty minutes each day thinking about getting bigger, being too small, or not being big enough. In addition, individuals with muscle dysmorphia check mirrors, on average, nine to thirteen times per day, compared with only three to five times per day for individuals who use the gym but do not have muscle dysmorphia. Although three to five times per day may seem high for individuals without muscle dysmorphia, it is important to consider that the weightlifting sections of most gyms have floor-to-ceiling mirrors on their walls. In this context, some degree of mirror checking is unavoidable. Finally, individuals with muscle dysmorphia weigh themselves, on average, four to five times per week (i.e. a bit more than every second day), while men who go to the gym but do not have muscle dysmorphia weigh themselves, on average, between once and twice per week. In summary, it is the cumulative amount of investment in the pursuit of a muscular body, measured in both time spent thinking and frequency of behaviours, that constitutes a key, necessary component of muscle dysmorphia.

Critically, however, for an adolescent to be diagnosed with muscle dysmorphia, the aforementioned investment in the pursuit of a muscular body *must* be accompanied by impairment in personal, social and/or academic functioning. In other words, it is entirely possible for an adolescent to be heavily involved in weight training or bodybuilding, frequently think and talk about bodybuilding, and buy and consume legal nutritional supplements, and *not* have muscle dysmorphia, so long as these investments of time and energy do not compromise their quality of life and ability to function as an individual, with others, and at school.

What constitutes 'impairment' in personal, social and academic functioning? As with the term 'preoccupied', the term 'impairment' is also subjective and prone to misinterpretation. Individuals with muscle dysmorphia often go to great lengths to hide or conceal their bodies, particularly in public places, including, for example, changing rooms, beaches and swimming pools. Individuals with muscle dysmorphia may wear extra clothing, even during hot weather, in an attempt to conceal their bodies. In one study, 88 per cent of men with muscle dysmorphia reported that they had worn heavy sweatshirts in the summer or refused to take their shirt off in public, due to the fear that someone would judge them as too small.[2] In comparison, of the thirty men who went to the gym but did not have muscle dysmorphia, not one admitted to doing this. These self-imposed limitations can place strain on a sufferer's relationships with friends and family. Strain on romantic relationships may also be evident. In the same study, 54 per cent of men with muscle dysmorphia reported that they had found themselves in an 'awkward sexual situation', compared with just 13 per cent of men who went to the gym but did not have muscle dysmorphia, presumably due to embarrassment, anxiety, or other negative feelings experienced as a result of appearing naked. In general, individuals with muscle dysmorphia report extreme functional impairment that directly results from their muscle dysmorphia, meaning that their thoughts and behaviours surrounding the pursuit of muscularity have a clear and sustained negative impact on their personal lives, social lives, school and/or job performance. Sometimes this impairment is not clear to the individual – only at the urging of others will they come to realise that their muscularity-focused thoughts and behaviours have begun to negatively affect their lives.

WHAT CAUSES MUSCLE DYSMORPHIA?

Muscle dysmorphia is complex and under-researched. Studies of muscle dysmorphia have, however, revealed putative risk factors that may increase the chances of an individual developing the disorder. It's important to keep in mind that an adolescent satisfying a risk factor, or even multiple risk factors, for muscle dysmorphia, is not indicative of that individual having muscle dysmorphia, nor can it substitute for a formal diagnosis of muscle dysmorphia made by a qualified health professional.

Body dissatisfaction: Being acutely unhappy with one's body shape and/or size is particularly common in muscle dysmorphia. *Professionals: for more information please visit the Generation Next website.*

History of an eating disorder: As previously discussed, there is considerable overlap between muscle dysmorphia and eating disorders. *Professionals: for more information please visit the Generation Next website.*

Escalating supplement use: Supplements include a variety of legal products and potions advertised to improve health, exercise performance, muscle synthesis, fat burning and boost testosterone, among other outcomes. Supplements vary considerably in safety, efficacy and cost. For example, protein powder is safe, effective and (relatively) cheap. Fears that excess protein consumption may cause kidney damage have proven to be largely unfounded. Only very few individuals with a genetic predisposition to kidney problems will experience health issues if they consume extremely high levels of protein. In addition, protein powders work, insofar as they help to build muscle. Whether adolescents *need* protein powder, however, depends on their diet (many people consume sufficient protein as part of their regular diet such that the addition of protein powder achieves little), and many dietitians would argue that consuming protein-rich whole foods is a better alternative, in general, to purchasing and consuming supplemental protein. The picture is less clear for other supplements, for example, testosterone boosters. *Professionals: for more information please visit the Generation Next website.*

Steroid use: Anabolic steroids are powerful drugs that are highly effective at building muscle – a property that makes them attractive to individuals with muscle dysmorphia. Estimates of the proportion of individuals with muscle dysmorphia who use steroids range from 40 to 50 per cent, compared with 6 to 14 per cent for men who attend the gym but do not have muscle dysmorphia. *Professionals: for more information please visit the Generation Next website.*

WHAT TO DO WHEN YOU OR SOMEONE YOU KNOW MAY HAVE MUSCLE DYSMORPHIA

Muscle dysmorphia should be diagnosed by a qualified mental health professional such as a psychologist or psychiatrist. As with all mental disorders, it is important to seek help early. This is so that, first, the disorder, if present, can be addressed before it becomes entrenched and more resistant to change, and, second, if the disorder is absent, then the anxiety and concerns surrounding the 'what-ifs' of a potential muscle dysmorphia diagnosis can be assuaged. The decision to seek help is often a challenging one to make because boys in particular are reluctant to admit to and discuss mental health concerns, especially those related to body image, which is often (mis)perceived as a 'girls-only problem'. Recent research indicates that this is manifestly untrue – most boys think about their physical appearance and body image to at least some degree and, indeed, a majority of Australian men are at least somewhat dissatisfied with their bodies. The act of seeking help may be made more difficult for boys because they tend to be more masculine than girls, and traditional ideas of masculinity and what it means to 'be a man' encourage emotional self-control, restricted emotional self-expression and emotional independence. Because none of these tenets of masculinity are particularly conducive to help seeking, it can take some convincing before a young boy or young man will take concrete steps to seek help. For parents, patience, compassion and tact will go a long way towards expediting this process.

The inconsistency in recognition of muscle dysmorphia reflects the paucity of research that has been conducted on the disorder. As a result, not all health professionals will be aware of, let alone understand, the complexities of muscle dysmorphia. General practitioners, including the family doctor, may not be aware of the disorder, and some discussion may need to take place about what muscle dysmorphia is (and what it isn't). Referral to a qualified mental health professional is the appropriate course of action in the event that muscle dysmorphia or a related mental disorder is suspected.

It is important to understand that there are few, if any, mental health professionals who specialise exclusively in muscle dysmorphia. Mental health professionals with expertise in treating eating disorders and/or body dysmorphic disorder are among the most likely to know of, and understand, muscle dysmorphia, and therefore are the most likely to be able to help. Expertise in eating disorders is desirable because of the considerable overlap between muscle dysmorphia and anorexia, and because a great deal of research on muscle dysmorphia is published in, and presented at, scholarly journals and conferences that are specific to eating disorders. For these reasons, a young person or their parents should request a referral to mental health professionals with expertise in eating disorders and/or body dysmorphic disorder. Do not be afraid to ask questions or make requests. Asking a mental health professional about their areas of expertise is a smart and acceptable strategy to ensure that they are up to speed on muscle dysmorphia. Similarly, asking a general practitioner to write a referral to a mental health professional with expertise in eating disorders is a smart and acceptable strategy to connect you or your child to an effective treatment solution as quickly as possible.

A mental health professional who makes a formal diagnosis of muscle dysmorphia will likely recommend mental health treatment. In turn, the treatment for muscle dysmorphia will likely take one of two forms: Cognitive Behavioural Therapy (CBT) or Family-Based Therapy (FBT).

POSSIBLE WARNING SIGNS OF MUSCLE DYSMORPHIA

- Feeling acutely unhappy with one's body shape and/or size, and muscles more specifically.
- Concealing one's body from others.
- Frequent mirror-checking and weighing.
- Frequently seeking reassurance from others in regard to one's body shape and/or size.
- Frequent negative self-directed comments about one's body shape and/or size.
- Rigid, strict and sustained dieting aimed at building muscle.
- Rigid, strict and sustained weight training aimed at building muscle.
- Feeling intense distress and/or anxiety as a result of disruptions to one's diet and/or weight training (e.g. an unexpected visit from a relative that prompts a spontaneous meal at a restaurant).
- Steroid use, positive intentions to use steroids, and/or positive beliefs about steroid use.
- Eating disorder behaviours, including bingeing and/or purging.
- Social withdrawal from friends and family.
- Loss of interest in activities other than dieting, exercise and bodybuilding.
- Declining school performance.
- Declining job performance.
- Continuing to lift weights despite physical pain and/or refusal to take time off from lifting weights in order to allow injuries to appropriately heal (i.e. the pain of lifting weights with an injury is preferable to the anxiety caused by not working out).

CBT for muscle dysmorphia involves challenging maladaptive or harmful beliefs surrounding body image, eating and exercise. Examples of maladaptive or harmful beliefs can include: 'If I can't be muscular then I'm worthless', 'I'll never get a girlfriend/boyfriend – nobody will ever love me if I don't work out', 'I'm a failure if I slip up on my diet', and 'Nobody will ever respect me because I'm scrawny/

fat'. These beliefs come in many shapes and forms and this list is not prescriptive. CBT challenges these beliefs with contravening evidence and attempts to create new beliefs and thoughts that are more firmly grounded in reality, do not induce intensely negative emotions, and which help to relax the rigidity surrounding body image, dieting and exercise. In addition, CBT challenges patterns of behaviour that both characterise and reinforce muscle dysmorphia, including, for example, compulsive weightlifting, mirror-checking, weighing, 'pinching', grabbing or otherwise checking one's body, seeking reassurance from others (e.g. 'Be honest – do I look scrawny in this singlet?') and steroid use. FBT is similar to CBT with the main exception being that the family unit is enlisted in treatment. Families, in conjunction with the mental health professional, are required to exert temporary control over their child's eating and exercise habits, until such a time that these habits have become normalised (i.e. no longer characteristic of muscle dysmorphia).

Evidence of effective treatments for muscle dysmorphia is extremely limited due to the little research on this condition. Given the substantial overlap between muscle dysmorphia and eating disorders, it is *likely* that CBT and FBT will be helpful for individuals with muscle dysmorphia. In a published case report, my colleague and I successfully conducted a course of FBT for an adolescent with muscle dysmorphia, achieving remission at the end of treatment. However, this single case report falls well short of providing a robust evidence base for treatment for muscle dysmorphia. Further, it is important to understand that even though CBT and FBT *do* work for eating disorders, they nevertheless are not effective for a substantial number of these individuals. For all these reasons, successful treatment for muscle dysmorphia relies, in part, on persistence, tenacity, resilience and a willingness to try alternatives if one treatment fails to work.

CAN MUSCLE DYSMORPHIA BE PREVENTED?

Prevention programmes designed specifically for muscle dysmorphia have not been trialled. Some schools in Australia have trialled prevention programmes for related disorders and likely risk factors for muscle dysmorphia, including eating disorders and body image dissatisfaction. A primary goal of these prevention programmes is to teach adolescents the skills and strategies they need to better manage their thoughts, feelings and beliefs surrounding body image, dieting, and exercise. There is some evidence that these programmes are effective for preventing the onset of eating disorders and body dissatisfaction, and, based on these successes, it is likely that adaptations of these programmes to specifically accommodate male body image and muscle dysmorphia would be effective in preventing the onset of muscle dysmorphia and related behaviours (e.g. steroid use).

WHAT CAN PARENTS DO TO HELP?

- Recognise and accept that boys growing up today are confronted by many of the same social pressures that have historically been levied at girls, and that boys thinking about their bodies and physical appearance is now the rule, not the exception.
- Tell your children that while it's okay that they think about how they look and that they put time and effort into their physical appearance, this must be *balanced* with *all the other important things in their lives*, including their friendships, school work, mental health, physical health and finances.
- Tell your children that they can talk to you about how they feel about their bodies and that you won't judge them for it. Avoid giving platitudes such as 'Don't even worry about it – girls don't like muscles anyway' and 'The gym is a waste of time – why not read a book instead?' Listen, validate, reassure and give well-meaning advice only in moderation.
- Aim for 'soft compromises'. For example, if your child is reluctant to speak to a health professional, you might try telling them that you'll make the appointment for two weeks from now, that you'll let them do most of the talking to the doctor, and that you won't bring it up between now and then

after they agree. This process can be extremely difficult – tact and patience are key.

- Recognise that you are already trying hard. Families with children with eating disorders often struggle immensely with the pressure of having a child with an eating disorder, and frequently report feeling like they have failed their child. It is critical to take a mental inventory and recognise that muscle dysmorphia is equally as complex as eating disorders, that its myriad causes are largely unknown, and that many other capable and kind-hearted parents have found themselves in the same unfortunate position. It is not at all your fault.

TAKE-HOME MESSAGES FOR PARENTS

- Muscle dysmorphia is the result of a societal trend – more and more boys are worried about their physical appearance, particularly their muscles.
- Both boys and girls can develop muscle dysmorphia. Girls who develop muscle dysmorphia are not weird or aberrant in any way (and neither are boys who develop anorexia).
- Encourage your sons and daughters to talk to you about how they feel about their bodies.
- Emphasise that everyone worries about their appearance some of the time and to some extent – the problem is that sometimes this worry can cross over a line from okay to not okay.
- Muscle dysmorphia should be diagnosed by a qualified health professional, and ideally a mental health professional with expertise in eating disorders.
- An adolescent can regularly go to the gym, buy and consume supplements, and discuss bodybuilding with their friends, and *not* have muscle dysmorphia. Muscle dysmorphia is relatively rare – don't jump the gun!
- Create an environment at home in which family members are encouraged to be open about their feelings – this will encourage your teen to speak up if they need to.

TAKE-HOME MESSAGES FOR TEACHERS AND SCHOOL COUNSELLORS/YOUTH WORKERS

- Explicitly telling boys that body image pressures on boys are the rule, not the exception, and that muscle dysmorphia is a body image condition akin to 'reverse anorexia', can provide a framework for how they think about their own bodies, exercise and training.
- Tell students that everyone worries about their physical appearance to some extent, and the fact that students engage in behaviours to improve their appearance is understandable (albeit not to be encouraged). The key message is that there is a line at which investment in appearance crosses over from okay to not okay and that this line is different depending on the person.

Author biography

Dr Scott Griffiths is a National Health and Medical Research Council (NHMRC) Research Fellow at the University of Melbourne. His research has attracted multiple awards and distinctions, including from the Australian Academy of Science, the Society for Mental Health Research, the Australian and New Zealand Academy of Eating Disorders, the North American Academy of Eating Disorders, and the University of Sydney.

www.psych.usyd.edu.au

See also:

Chapter 4: Anxiety in Young People
Chapter 5: Depression in Young People
Chapter 6: Understanding Self-harm
Chapter 7: Suicide and Attempted Suicide
Chapter 12: Understanding Eating Disorders in Young People
Chapter 13: Excessive Dieting and Exercise
Chapter 14: Anorexia Nervosa
Chapter 15: Bulimia and Binge Eating
Chapter 17: Fostering a Positive Body Image

Recommended websites:

Body Dysmorphic Disorder Foundation: bddfoundation.org
Mind: www.mind.org.uk
NHS: nhs.uk/conditions/body-dysmorphia
The Mix: www.themix.org.uk/your-body/fitness-and-diet

Further reading:

Cafri, G, Olivardia, R & Thompson, JK 2008, 'Symptom characteristics and psychiatric comorbidity among males with muscle dysmorphia', *Comprehensive Psychiatry*, vol. 49, no. 4, pp 374–379.

Hitzeroth, V, Wessels, C, Zungu Dirwayi, N, Oosthuizen, P & Stein, DJ 2001, 'Muscle dysmorphia: A South African sample', *Psychiatry and Clinical Neurosciences*, vol. 55, pp 521–523.

Olivardia, R, Pope, HG & Hudson, J 2000, 'Muscle dysmorphia in male weightlifters: A case-control study', *American Journal of Psychiatry*, vol. 157, no. 8, pp 1291–1296.

Pope, HG Jnr, Phillips, KA, Olivardio, R 2002, *The Adonis Complex*, Simon & Schuster, New York.

For more online resources visit:
generationnext.com.au/handbook

17. FOSTERING A POSITIVE BODY IMAGE

Professor Susan Paxton & Dr Siân McLean

This chapter will provide an overview of important influences on body image in adolescence. Readers will gain an understanding of the role of peers and media, and approaches to prevent these influences from having a negative effect on body image.

INTRODUCTION

Body image refers to how a person thinks, feels and behaves in relation to their body. Often it is assumed that body image refers specifically to a person's body size; although body size frequently has an influence on body image, body image itself relates to how a person evaluates their own body. Because of the cultural norms for, and emphasis on, physical attractiveness in western societies, this evaluation typically focuses on weight and shape in females, and muscularity and leanness in males.

Body image may be thought of as falling on a continuum from positive to negative body image. A person at the positive end of the continuum is happy with their body and accepts it despite perceived faults. These attitudes build confidence and a positive connection with the body, described as embodiment. At the negative end of the continuum, however, a person feels intense dislike, loathing, shame and embarrassment about their appearance. In research into body image, these negative emotions and attitudes are frequently described as body image concerns or body dissatisfaction. This type of terminology can make it sound as though body dissatisfaction is fairly unimportant. But body dissatisfaction may be so intense and painful that it has an extremely negative impact on a person's life.

Body dissatisfaction may cause great distress and reduced quality of life. In addition, body dissatisfaction is important to understand because it contributes to the development of other problems in males and females, including low self-esteem and depressive symptoms, lower physical activity, increased smoking and sexual risk-taking, use of unhealthy and extreme weight-loss or muscle-gain measures, and the development of severe clinical eating disorders.

Body image attitudes are formed during childhood and research shows that about 50 per cent of eight- to eleven-year-old girls and 40 per cent of eight- to eleven-year-old boys think a lot about being thinner. However, research has mostly focused on body image in adolescents as this is the time when body dissatisfaction has its biggest impact. Consistent with overseas studies, a 2015 survey conducted by Mission Australia of nearly 19 000 fifteen- to nineteen-year-old adolescents found that 37.4 per cent of females and 13.1 per cent of males described themselves as extremely or very concerned about their body image. Once established, body-image concerns frequently continue into adulthood and midlife, and continue to have a negative impact on wellbeing.

SIGNS THAT A YOUNG PERSON IS EXPERIENCING BODY DISSATISFACTION

- Preoccupation with weight, shape or size.
- Body weight, shape or size being very important for self-worth.
- Frequent weighing or checking body size.
- Avoiding social activities that may bring attention to appearance.
- Feeling a very strong need to control weight, shape or size.
- Excessive amounts of time spent exercising, including weight training, especially when ill or injured, or feeling guilty for not exercising.

RISK FACTORS FOR THE DEVELOPMENT
OF BODY DISSATISFACTION

Exploration into risk factors that contribute to the development of body dissatisfaction has been an important area of research. The main reason for this is the underlying theory that if influential risk factors are reduced, or the action of the risk factors blocked, then the pathway to developing body dissatisfaction will be interrupted. This knowledge about the pathways to body dissatisfaction can therefore inform effective prevention interventions. A number of risk factors have been identified that may broadly be categorised as biological, individual, psychological and sociocultural factors.

Biological risk factors, including genetic factors, are very likely to play a role. However, as we have little understanding about how these can be modified, they have not been a focus for prevention. A larger body size also increases risk of body dissatisfaction. This is not because there is an intrinsic link between larger body size and body dissatisfaction, but because larger body sizes are viewed negatively within our culture. Individual temperament and psychological variables including low self-esteem, depressive symptoms and perfectionism also increase risk of body dissatisfaction, so building a child's confidence during childhood will foster positive body image as they grow older.

Sociocultural factors for body dissatisfaction include environments that increase pressure to conform to the narrow appearance ideals of thinness for females and muscularity and leanness for males that are present in western cultures. The risk factors increase the importance placed on appearance and achieving appearance ideals, and individuals may come to believe that their own value as a person is dependent on meeting these ideals. This is known as internalisation of appearance ideals. Internalisation of appearance ideals increases the extent to which one compares one's own body with others and, as comparisons are typically made with others who have more of a desired quality, body dissatisfaction ensues.

Risk environments include families in which there is a high value placed on appearance ideals. It is therefore important to assist families to create a positive body image environment for their children in which there is acceptance of diversity and focus on non-appearance qualities of children. However, two other sociocultural influences are important to consider as they may be modified by school or community interventions: appearance-focused media and appearance-focused peer environments.

MEDIA INFLUENCE ON BODY IMAGE

Media has been the focus of much research on risk factors for body dissatisfaction. The representation of females and males in media regularly shows people who are thinner and who are more muscular than average people in society. The media also creates social norms for appearance by portraying people who meet appearance ideals in a positive manner and portraying people who do not meet appearance ideals in a negative manner.

Regular viewing of this type of media creates the impression that it is normal for women to be very thin and normal for men to be very muscular. Furthermore, the impression viewers receive from media, particularly advertising by the weight-loss industry, is that it should be easy to attain an appearance consistent with sociocultural ideals. However, the extremes of thinness and muscularity shown in media represent body sizes that are unrealistic for most people to attain.

It is also important to recognise that the presentation of both female and male bodies in media focuses on the body as an object to be viewed by others, rather than focusing on the body as an active agent where function is more important than appearance. This type of presentation further reinforces appearance ideals as valuable to attain.

In the media, people whose appearance is consistent with ideals – that is thin and attractive for females and muscular and lean for males – are typically shown as being happy, having fun, being successful in careers and social relationships, and powerful. In contrast, the media typically shows people who do not meet appearance ideals, particularly in relation to their weight, as less intelligent, more unfriendly, as having fewer friends or romantic relationships, and more likely to be the 'bad' character, than are people who are of average weight or underweight. It should be noted that males who are smaller than the muscular appearance ideal can also be stigmatised in the media.

These messages are present in all types of media, including magazines, television, music videos, animated cartoons directed at children, video games for adolescents and adults, and social media. Thus, all forms of media create social norms that influence the type of appearance that is seen to be attractive, desirable and valuable to attain.

When these ideals are internalised by individuals as personal standards which they aspire to attain, and they compare how they look with the internalised standards, body dissatisfaction occurs. The individual feels inferior to the standards they wish to live up to.

Research has shown that when people view idealised media images, they are likely to experience increased body dissatisfaction. This is more likely to occur if they have internalised appearance ideals and if they have a tendency to compare how they look with others. It has also been shown that the more people view media that has a focus on appearance, including things like watching television soap operas or music videos, the greater their levels of body image concerns.

Social media is highly visual and interactive, and entails active engagement by users, rather than passive viewing. Social media use is potentially problematic for body image due to the high focus on appearance in social media content and due to the frequency and amount of time spent engaging with various social media platforms by young people and adolescents. According to the Australian Bureau of Statistics, in Australia in 2013, 97 per cent of adolescents are internet users, and of these 90 per cent use the internet for social networking. Further, studies of adolescent girls indicate they typically spend one and a half to two hours on these sites a day and have on average over 200 social network 'friends'.

As with traditional media, social media reinforces thin and muscular ideals for appearance through repeated presentations of these ideals, and also through the activities of social media users which reinforce the perceived rewards from achieving appearance ideals. For example, through Facebook, Instagram, Pinterest or other platforms, users can choose to follow celebrities or follow hashtags, which are used for categorising content according to common themes or interests. This has the effect of altering individuals' social media environments by delivering constant updates on personal devices in relation to the followed celebrity or hashtag. Depending on what is followed, this has the potential to create a social media environment that is saturated with appearance-ideal content which in turn enhances the likelihood of experiencing body image concerns.

In relation to rewards from meeting appearance ideals, social media enables very tangible and observable feedback about one's appearance in the form of collecting 'likes' from one's own photo posting. Further, social media engagement creates pressure on individuals to post 'selfies', which present their appearance in the best light. Research has shown that frequent engagement in social media photo-based activities, manipulation of photos through application of filters or photo editing techniques, or concern about selecting appropriate photos to post are associated with body image concerns. Although these activities may not cause body dissatisfaction, it is likely that they contribute to the maintenance of body image concerns. Thus, intervention regarding these activities that enhance focus on appearance has the potential to reduce body dissatisfaction.

MEDIA LITERACY AND BODY IMAGE

As well as understanding the role of risk factors, it can also be very helpful to understand the ways in which other factors can protect against the development of body image concerns. For example, a person who is media literate has the ability to think critically about media, to evaluate the plausibility of media content, and to understand the creative processes behind it. Research has shown that when people have higher media literacy skills they are less negatively affected by viewing media that promotes the thin ideal or the muscular ideal appearance. They are also less likely to internalise appearance ideals or compare their own appearance to how others look.

People who are media literate recognise the persuasive intent of media producers. In relation to the presentation of appearance ideals, this may mean understanding that media are constructed through digital editing and use extreme ideals to sell products by promoting an aspirational image. If an understanding of these tactics is reached, people may be less inclined to accept that media appearance ideals are desirable as they perceive them to be unrealistic and less self-relevant, and constructed by media and advertising companies to exploit the vulnerabilities of viewers.

A further way media-literate individuals may be protected from media is by questioning the truth of media that stigmatises different body shapes and sizes. When people become aware of and examine the weight bias in media, they tend to reject media that sends those messages. They may choose to disengage from particular magazines, television shows or social media sites, or actively engage in creating new media content to displace unhelpful or stigmatising messages.

PEER INFLUENCES ON BODY IMAGE

There has been increasing recognition that peers and friends play an important role in providing an environment which either supports positive body image or increases the risk for the development of body image concerns. Research shows that friendship groups tend to share similar levels of body satisfaction or dissatisfaction partly due to the influence of friends on each other and partly due to young people selecting friends who are more like themselves in attitudes and interests. Therefore, it is helpful to consider how peers and friends influence each other so that they come to adopt similar beliefs about the importance of meeting appearance ideals.

Appearance conversations: An important way of communicating appearance norms is through peer appearance conversations. In girls, these conversations frequently involve wanting to be thinner, feeling fat, needing to lose weight, weight-loss methods, the appearance of celebrities, clothes, fashion and photos posted online. They may take place in face-to-face settings or online. In boys, appearance conversations are more likely to include conversations about working out at the gym, sports training, muscle development, supplements or dietary strategies to lose fat and also gain muscle mass. Through these discussions, young people communicate to others the perceived importance of meeting cultural appearance ideals and internalise shared norms. In addition, they increase body comparisons among peers, especially with others perceived to have more of the qualities desired than they do. Body dissatisfaction, and use of unhealthy weight loss or muscle gain strategies frequently follow. It is important to note, however, that in some friendship groups there are relatively few appearance conversations but, rather, there is discussion of other shared interests. These environments are associated with more positive body image and less disordered eating.

Appearance teasing and criticism: Another way in which peers may influence body image and eating behaviours is through appearance-related teasing, criticism or rejection. Adolescence is a developmental period in which there is a particularly high need to be accepted and included by friends, so it is not surprising that being teased and rejected, especially in relation to appearance, increases negative thoughts and feelings directed towards one's own body.

Peer body dissatisfaction, dieting and importance of appearance: Adolescents may also learn that meeting appearance ideals is either essential to being a valuable person or not by observing the attitudes and behaviours of their friends. Even in early primary school, girls' perceived peer desire for thinness has been shown to predict the later development of body dissatisfaction, while in adolescence friends' dieting predicts the development of dieting and unhealthy weight control behaviours.

Friends and social media: The nature of peer and friendship environments has changed greatly with the advent of social media and social networking sites. These environments extend friendship interactions from face to face to online interactions in a highly engaging and intense way. Social media friendship environments have the potential to have a particularly strong influence on body image as they are typically highly visual and sharing photos of the self and comparing with others' self-photo posts are often central activities.

In relation to selfie posting, there is a high expectation and hope that if a photo is posted, friends will 'like' the photo and post favourable comments. Interestingly, 'likes' have greater currency than positive comments. Research has found that adolescent girls' perception of their status within their peer group was highly dependent on the number of likes received for photos and comparison with the numbers of likes received by peers. Receiving fewer likes than expected, or fewer than peers' – particularly rivals for popularity within the peer group – was found to be associated with greater feelings of self-consciousness and doubts about self-worth.

Not surprisingly, adolescents may spend a great deal of time posing for a photo, selecting a photo or manipulating a photo to be shared on a social networking site. However, there is the possibility that friends will not 'like' or not comment on posted photos, which is immediately interpreted as not liking the photo or, more generally, the appearance of the poster. For adolescents, lack of response to social media photo posts represents disapproval by others. Especially for teenagers who already lack confidence in themselves or their body, this has as big an impact as face-to-face exclusions. In addition, there is the possibility of specifically negative comments about a posted photo, which are as painful as face-to-face criticism. Receiving negative comments about social media updates contributes to greater weight and shape concerns.

HARNESSING PEER INTERACTIONS AND MEDIA LITERACY

Peer interactions and media literacy can be harnessed to create positive environments that reduce pressure to conform to narrow appearance ideals of thinness for females and muscularity and leanness for males.

This can be achieved in two ways. First, adolescents can actively change their own environments so as to create an environment with fewer appearance ideal pressures and greater appreciation of non-appearance-related qualities. Second, they may be assisted to reduce engagement with peer and media risk factors in their environment over which they do have control, and to develop skills to counter or cope with the negative pressures they face from aspects of these environments over which they don't.

Interventions that have been shown to improve body image and reduce risk factors have typically been school-based, with students attending three to eight lessons that explore environmental appearance pressures and ways that these can be counteracted. It's essential that all activities are highly interactive and engaging and allow students to reach their own conclusions about media and peer influences rather than being told in a didactic manner what the problems are, as young people are much more likely to believe what they discover for themselves than what they are told. Useful intervention resources are described at the end of this chapter.

Typically, the first step in countering media and peer influences is to raise awareness in students of the nature of our society's appearance ideals and the body image and self-esteem problems that these ideals can cause. Additional exploration of the sources of pressure to conform to these ideals can lead to the identification of roles of media, peers and family.

Once young people are aware that they live in environments that promote unrealistic and unhealthy appearance ideals, a deeper exploration of the source of these pressures is important. Building media literacy is an especially important approach. Students learn to critique media images and to examine commercial interests behind idealised media appearance images and pressures coming from advertising, fashion and celebrity culture. This helps to clarify the reason these ideals are so strongly promoted. Interactive activities in which students observe the creation of advertising images highlight the unreality of the images and the wide range of make-up, photographic strategies and digital manipulation that go into the media images we see. Projects in which students are encouraged to take an activist stance against unreal or unhealthy advertising – for example, to write to a magazine editor to complain of a highly idealised image – can be particularly helpful.

Another approach to reducing internalisation of appearance ideals is known as the cognitive dissonance approach to intervention. This is one in which students engage in activities in which they challenge appearance ideals. For example, they may create presentations or posters that present arguments describing why striving to meet unrealistic appearance ideals and valuing yourself according to appearance is not a good thing as it leads to body image concerns and lower self-esteem.

Exploration of friendship environments can also help students identify and understand aspects in their own social world that can amplify body image concerns. It's important that adolescents understand the power of appearance conversations (e.g. talking about things you don't like about your body or dieting) in creating and building body image concerns in friendship groups. Problems associated with appearance teasing and the negative impact of appearance-based victimisation and weight bias can also be explored. Students can role play ways to change appearance conversations if they hear them among their friends and discuss ways to challenge appearance teasing among friends. It's useful to provide opportunities for adolescents to consider what they truly value in their friends as these are very seldom appearance-based qualities. Importantly, these discoveries can provide students with ideas about how they can change their own environment to create friendship environments that support positive body image.

To date, programmes specifically addressing online peer relationships and coping with the social media world have not yet been evaluated. It's likely, though, that providing an opportunity for young people to critique both commercial and personal postings made on social media will provide additional coping strategies for young people in this new appearance-focused environment.

In addition, others, from celebrities to close friends, typically like to post images of themselves that show themselves and their lives in the best light. Often images have been posted that have been taken at particular angles or in particular settings, and are also manipulated in a range of ways so that the image is far from realistic. With this understanding, adolescents can consider whether these are appropriate targets for comparison. Further, young people can be encouraged to consider whether engaging in this online appearance culture has any negative impact on them and if so, they can explore ways of coping with these pressures from social media.

TAKE-HOME MESSAGES FOR PARENTS

Be aware that even though body dissatisfaction is common, it does not mean that it's harmless. Do not confuse body dissatisfaction with vanity. Body dissatisfaction can be very distressing and lead to the development of other problems.

If you think that your child is experiencing body dissatisfaction, it is important to intervene. Ask open, inquisitive questions. Show respect for children's beliefs by validating their concerns without reinforcing unrealistic appearance ideals.

Help your child to have a balanced perception of their self-worth by increasing their focus on qualities other than appearance. Praising your child for their enjoyment of and achievements in areas unrelated to appearance will assist with this.

If your child is feeling distressed or is engaging in unhealthy behaviours to control their weight, shape or size, seek professional assistance.

Parents can provide a positive body image environment for young people by:

- Modelling a positive attitude to their own and others' bodies:
  - Speak positively about your own body.
  - Demonstrate acceptance of different body shapes and sizes in others.
  - Do not equate personal characteristics in people according to their body size.

- Not criticising or teasing (or allowing others to do so) your child's appearance, even as a joke.
- Encouraging your child to accept their body:
  - Help your child to focus on the functions of their body and what it can achieve.

TAKE-HOME MESSAGES FOR TEACHERS AND SCHOOL COUNSELLORS/YOUTH WORKERS

Teachers can promote a positive school environment for body image by:

- Intervening in peer interactions and engagement with media that promote pressure to attain appearance ideals by:
  - Diverting appearance conversations that reinforce the importance of appearance ideals.
  - Not permitting weight-related teasing/jokes.
  - Encouraging critique of media or current events that reinforce thinness and muscularity appearance ideals or disparage larger body sizes, for example, media commentary on the appearance of high-profile women.
  - Delivering an evidence-based classroom body image programme.
- Amending school policies that may contribute to body dissatisfaction. For example, class activities involving weighing and measuring students should be omitted from the curriculum.
- Ensuring school bullying policies address weight bias and appearance-based teasing.
- Ensuring all uniforms, including sports uniforms, cause no embarrassment for students.
- Recognising the presence of body dissatisfaction and referring to school wellbeing or counselling teams.

Authors' biographies

Professor Susan Paxton is a Professor in the School of Psychology and Public Health, La Trobe University. She is a Director of The Butterfly Foundation and past President of the Academy for Eating Disorders. In recognition of her research, she was awarded the 2013 Academy for Eating Disorders Leadership in Research Award.

Dr Siân McLean is Lecturer in Psychology in the College of Health and Biomedicine at Victoria University and an Honorary Research Fellow in the School of Psychology and Public Health, La Trobe University. She is highly experienced in school-based prevention and research investigating the role of media literacy as a protective factor in the development of body dissatisfaction.

See also:
Chapter 4: Anxiety in Young People
Chapter 5: Depression in Young People
Chapter 6: Understanding Self-harm
Chapter 7: Suicide and Attempted Suicide
Chapter 12: Understanding Eating Disorders in Young People
Chapter 13: Excessive Dieting and Exercise
Chapter 14: Anorexia Nervosa
Chapter 15: Bulimia and Binge Eating

Recommended websites:
National Centre for Eating Disorders: eating-disorders.org.uk
The Mix: www.ncsyes.co.uk/themix/body-image-facts
Eating Disorder Hope: www.eatingdisorderhope.com/information/body-image
The Be Real Campaign: www.berealcampaign.co.uk

For more online resources visit:
generationnext.com.au/handbook

RESILIENCE, POSITIVE PSYCHOLOGY AND A HEALTHY LIFESTYLE

What is Resilience and How to Do It   281

Harnessing the Minecraft Mindset for Success   292

Using Positive Psychology   306

Food, Mood and Mental Health   323

Understanding the Teenage Brain   335

Online Time Management   349

18. WHAT IS RESILIENCE AND HOW TO DO IT

Andrew Fuller

Resilience is the capacity to call upon the resources around you and within you to flexibly respond to whatever life throws at you. Resilience is also the creative and innovative process of creating opportunities to allow you to express your potential. This chapter will help you build resilience into your everyday life.

INTRODUCTION

Imagine you have just one chance. You are with a young person and you have just one chance to help them see that their life could be different.

We are in precisely that situation right now. We have a chance to help you to shift your perspectives about the possibility of change. You need to understand how change can occur rapidly for yourself before you can help others to do the same.

Often when we work with young people we have just one chance to make a difference. Disaffected young people are not especially enamoured with what older people have to tell them. Many are so used to a world of digital distractedness that lengthy conversations are experienced as tiresome and dull.

While change in people's lives is often seen as planned or painstaking, research on resilience and life trajectories for my book *Life: A Guide* showed that people's life patterns can and do shift both suddenly and dramatically.

The changes that occur in most people's lives are both rapid and pervasive. Seismic shifts in awareness occur. People change jobs, roles, schools, relationships and themselves in the flick of a moment. Just as episodes of trauma can shift the direction of life, so can times of positive growth and experience. People can transform and reinvent their lives.

You may have experienced this personally. You may have left a conversation or an encounter irrevocably altered. Your worldview expanded. The pathway to a new way of living opened before you.

There may be in your history or in your family's history times when circumstances shifted rapidly. In those moments the presence of resilience is lifesaving.

It is like the old story about a client who experienced a life-changing session with a psychologist and asked them, 'How long did it take you learn to do that?' The reply was, 'It took me five minutes to say it and twenty years to learn what to say.' Change in life can occur rapidly but it often has had years of small practices that allow the change to occur.

To transform our futures, we have to first transform ourselves.

THE OPPORTUNITY OF A LIFETIME

We have the chance of a lifetime to build the habits of resilience in young people. Resilience takes tough times and creates out of them great futures.

We know that our brains are shaped by our experiences. We also know that many of our behaviours are patterned and fairly habitual. We further know that under pressure, anxiety, and trauma, we act based on our patterns or habits to survive.

The development of resilience is more than just shifting people's thinking. It is about developing habits and practices that can be called upon in times of uncertainty and challenge. These practices also improve our everyday lives.

While rapid changes do occur in people's lives, they usually have a prelude. Most positive changes are the culmination of a series of little habits that have built themselves into practices that burst through as a positive change in life.

FROM SURVIVING TO THRIVING

Essentially, resilience is the capacity to call upon the resources around you and within you to flexibly respond to whatever life throws at you. Resilience is also the creative and innovative process of creating opportunities to allow you to express your potential.

Resilience enables us to endure the hard times and to capitalise on the good times so we can unlock the genius within ourselves.

PRACTISING THE ART OF RESILIENCE

Life is an improvisational art. At times we need to shape and reshape ourselves to bring the best of life into view. Sometimes we can do this on the spur of the moment but mostly it is best if we incorporate resilience-building practices into our everyday life.

The following practices are small acts that all of us can incorporate into our everyday lives to build resilience. These practices can also be used by young people to shape their brains and their lives. Let's call them resilience practices.

Resilience Practice One – Connect to others

Deepening our relationships with family, friends and even strangers builds resilience. The quality of our relationships powerfully determines the quality of our lives.

There may be people who you like or love but haven't had the chance to catch up with. Make a practice of staying in touch with the people you value.

People like people who like them. Welcome people into your life. Take on the practice of telling people that you like and appreciate them.

Find places and people who value what you have to offer. What is appreciated appreciates.

Stay away from places and people who do not seem to appreciate you or what you have to offer. Don't bother to blame them. Not everyone likes you or the things that you like. Don't blame yourself. You don't need everyone to like you.

Resilience Practice Two – Connect to yourself

Inscribed on the Temple of the Oracle in Delphi was 'know thyself'. Self-awareness means taking the time to get to know yourself. The whole box and dice – the faults, the foibles and the flaws just as much as the strengths.

Take some time each day to get to know yourself. Give yourself a check-up from the neck up:

- How am I feeling today?
- What am I enjoying?
- What is bothering me?
- What can I do to change that?

We all need to regularly de-traumatise ourselves. We all carry some wounds of trauma with us. These come from times when we felt overwhelmed and scared, and didn't process what was happening well enough to really understand it. These are often times when we don't look after ourselves, gain weight or feel exhausted.

If you find this hard to identify with, think about the times your reaction to something seems out of proportion to the circumstances, and start there.

While sitting quietly reflecting on events, writing, painting, dancing or singing about past traumas will help, you can only really process trauma in relationship with someone else.

Looking inwards and reflecting on life helps guide us about what we really want and value. Notice your energy patterns. What enlivens or excites you? What tires or bores you?

Find your creative spark or your passion. Ask yourself, what would you do if you knew you couldn't fail?

Resilience Practice Three – Develop
your sense of belonging

Our sense of belonging is a profoundly powerful creator of resilience. Think about where you have a sense of belonging. For many of us, there are special people, friends, family members who we feel we belong with. For others there are workplaces, teams, causes or clubs. Other people can add beaches, farms, cities, parks or holiday destinations to the list of places they belong.

We also belong to ourselves and the way we go about living our lives. This is why having practices that pattern themselves into habits creates the foundation of our lives.

Resilience Practice Four – Shift your radar

We are what we notice. In the average day we perceive over 7000 different things, feelings, ideas and sensations. We can't process all of those 7000 perceptions so we select some of them to make sense of. By making sense of those perceptions, we create a story of our day that helps us to understand what has been happening.

Our understanding of how our day has been is a story we create from the perceptions we have selected. You might have noticed this. You might have had days when it seems nothing goes right. You might have had other days when you've felt nothing could go wrong. Of course you've also had days that were a mixture.

By consciously deciding to pay attention to the good things that occur to us, we increase the balance of good to bad days. The main way of doing this is to be appreciative or grateful of the small things that happen in each day.

This doesn't mean that you blind yourself to bad things. Unwavering optimism can be sheer folly. Positive thinking alone can lead to despair when it is not realised. At the same time, focusing on faults and failures can lead to passivity and disempowerment.

It is possible to notice the good and the bad in the world and make the choice to use the magnifying glass on goodness.

Resilience Practice Five – Be where you are

Concentration, awareness, presence and mindfulness are all about the same thing: being where you are right now.

All psychological problems have an aspect of distractedness about them. If we become depressed we are often preoccupied by the past and regrets or shame. If we are anxious we often spend our time dreading future events. Welcome what is.

It is important to learn how to let the past be exactly what it is – past.

Acknowledge it, take from it, honour it, but don't let the worst parts of the past dictate your future. Similarly, rather than dreading the future, create it. As James Thurber once said, 'let us not look back in anger or forward in fear but around in awareness'.

In a world of distraction, concentration is hard to gain and easy to lose.

Practise taking time to be here.

Resilience Practice Six – Be hopeful

Hope is a powerful protector against despair. To lose hope is to lose your faith in the future. To lose hope is to lose trust in yourself.

In a world that values rankings and judgements and hard-edged cynicism, it takes courage to be hopeful. Being hopeful means you risk being labelled as naive or, worse, privileged and blind to the pains of others.

Hope is an act of courage that allows adaptation, creativity and opportunity. Any effective change in the world is an example of hope overtaking despair.

Behind every success is a series of failures. This is why failure and vulnerability are essential to our development as people. It is by embracing and learning from them that we can become resilient. What enables all of us to persist in the face of failure is hope.

Facing adversity, setbacks and failure enables resilience. Hope shifts us from broken-heartedness to whole-heartedness. In the thousands of people's lives that I have mapped, almost all followed a time of harsh adversity with sustained positive growth. These people didn't *feel* hopeful – they chose to *be* hopeful and made plans accordingly.

As Emily Dickinson once said, 'hope inspires the good to reveal itself'.

Resilience Practice Seven – Positive relationships

Follow the golden rule: treat other people as you would like to be treated yourself. This means being kind and respectful, and also being prepared to forgive rather than blaming others when mistakes are made.

Some people treat others well but are harshly self-critical, feeling inept and cringe-worthy. Apply the golden rule to yourself: treat yourself as well as you treat others.

Even if you are not especially sociable, broaden your social connections. Whenever you can, strike up conversations with people who are different from you. Find people you disagree with and understand them.

Resilience Practice Eight – Empowerment

Empowerment shifts people from 'No, I can't' to 'Yes, I can'. It is the basis of a learning mindset. Empowerment helps us to overcome our setbacks and to remain resilient in times of challenge.

One day you will discover that you are the leader you have been waiting for and start to work towards the changes you want to see happen.

Many people only express a small portion of their capabilities. They never really unlock their inner genius.

One of the ways to increase your sense of empowerment is to take on an even bigger job than the one you currently do. You might be a student, a teacher, a tradesperson or a professional but you can also take on a bigger job of powerfully changing something in the world. This might be to take on increasing happiness in the world or reducing poverty or increasing beauty. Find a job worthy of you and put energy into making it happen.

Resilience Practice Nine – Stretch your mind

Take yourself on mind-stretching and heart-opening adventures. Build your curiosity and your creativity.

If you get scared of getting things wrong, you won't try new things. If you don't try new things, you become bored and boring. Life becomes mundane, dull and routine.

Plan to do things you have never done before. Quirky adventures don't have to take a lot of time or money but they do take some thought and planning. Plan to go somewhere you've never been before or do something you have never done before. Don't settle for anything less than an interesting life.

Resilience Practice Ten – Sharpen your social skills

The acquisition of social skills powerfully protects against substance abuse.

One of the really simple ways to be a good friend to someone is to decide that you are lucky to know them.

Gaining brief eye contact with people communicates interest and trust. One simple way to do this is to mentally remind yourself to notice the colour of other people's eyes as you say hello to them.

One of the ways to live an interesting life is to talk to people who are different from you. Getting to know people from different countries and backgrounds will enrich your life and stretch your ideas.

FIVE VALUES THAT STAND OUT AND FEATURE IN QUALITY RELATIONSHIPS

Trust – trust others and be trustworthy.

Forgiveness – when mistakes are made, forgive yourself and others.

Integrity – be who you say you are and do what you say you will do.

Hope – build hope in the world.

Compassion – compassion is empathy on steroids. Empathy is seeing another's plight; compassion is being prepared to do something about it.

Resilience Practice Eleven – Clarify your values

Values are the positions we take that form the basis of our lives. They are what we stand for. Values don't shift according to circumstances or from moment to moment. They help us to be sure of ourselves.

Resilience Practice Twelve – Positive identity

Resilience is more about completeness and wholeness than happiness.

Taking the time to discover the treasures within you and to nourish and develop them is work that can take a lifetime. This requires times of reflection to develop self-knowledge.

Only you can occupy the corner of creation that is yours. When you take the time to develop your identity, your presence, your creativity and your energies come alive.

Summon the courage within you to explore and broaden your search for your passions. Take the risk of trying things out and seeing if they work for you. Too many people miss out on the great opportunities of life by pre-judging them as not worth investigating. Have a go.

As Howard Thurman put it, 'Don't ask what the world needs. Ask what makes you come alive, and go do it. Because what the world needs is people who have come alive.' Create a powerfully positive identity by making yourself come alive.

Resilience Practice Thirteen – Boundaries and expectations

Aim high, work hard and play hard. Do the tough stuff. Expect the best for yourself and want the best for others.

Challenge yourself. Take at least one area to develop a passion or a discipline in. Apply yourself to that area with devotion.

Humility is not about making yourself small, it is about readiness to find goodness and surprise and worth in people.

Resilience Practice Fourteen – Be your own health consultant

This doesn't mean doing a medical degree or consulting Dr Google over every ache and pain. It does mean seeking out the best, most qualified sources of information and acting upon them to increase your own wellbeing.

Seek out health expertise when you need it and also take your health seriously by completing your **MEDS**:

- **M**editation – find some place for calm for each day.
- **E**xercise – get your heart rate up a few times a week.
- **D**iet – use your pantry to increase your health.
- **S**leep – one of the most powerful ways to reduce stress and depression, increase memory and learning, build energy, slow ageing and lose weight is to sleep well.

Resilience Practice Fifteen – Adopt a guardian angel

As much as you look after your own health, don't simply rely on yourself. As you are immersed in your own life, there are times when you will be so busy you forget to look after yourself. Ask one or two people to act as guardian angels to you. These are people who you ask to tell you if you look stressed or weary or overwhelmed. Let them know you won't be offended. In fact, let them know you will take steps to look after yourself based on their feedback.

Resilience Practice Sixteen – Love

Love is contagious. Love more than is reasonable to do so. We live in a world that is impoverished in its vocabulary. The Persians had fifty-two words describing different types of love; we, of course, have one. We have no words to help us to realise our love of friends, beauty, the land we live in, the sea, animals, nature, music, art, family, our purpose and ourselves.

By focusing on the external forms of desire and love we lose something very important. We lose the ability for people to look within themselves for nourishment, energy and solace. We risk having people who are dependent, focused on external distractions and entertainments, and not as fully formed as people who value their own uniqueness.

By taking the time to celebrate and love the person you are and delight and love the people around you, you help others to love well, and if you can do that, you change the world.

Author biography

Andrew Fuller is a clinical psychologist and the author of many bestselling books that have been translated into twenty languages. These include *Life: A Guide – what to expect in each seven year stage*, *Tricky Teens*, *From Surviving to Thriving – Promoting Mental Health in Young People*, *Tricky Kids*, *Raising Real People*, *The Brain Based Learning E-manual*, and *Tricky People*. Andrew is a director of Resilient Youth.

www.andrewfuller.com.au

See also:
Chapter 19: Harnessing the Minecraft Mindset for Success
Chapter 20: Using Positive Psychology
Chapter 21: Food, Mood and Mental Health
Chapter 22: Understanding the Teenage Brain

Recommended website:
www.gov.uk/government/uploads/system/uploads/attachment_data/file/355766/
Review2_Resilience_in_schools_health_inequalities.pdf

For more online resources visit:
generationnext.com.au/handbook

19. HARNESSING THE MINECRAFT MINDSET FOR SUCCESS

Dan Haesler

This chapter will explore why Minecraft is so engaging for young (and older) children, and what parents, teachers and perhaps employers can learn from gaming mechanics to improve outcomes for young people.

INTRODUCTION

Read the newspapers or scan your social media feed, it won't be long before you come across an article lamenting the amount of time young people spend playing video games, how they've become disconnected from the 'real world', and how in many cases – despite not being officially recognised as such – video gaming could be seen as an 'addiction'.

But have you ever wondered why it is kids will fail over and over again at a video game and keep coming back for more, but only need to fail once or twice in class before giving up?

And just why do kids become agoraphobic when a new game hits the market?

Some research[1] would suggest that the average gamer in Australia is thirty-three years old and 47 per cent of gamers in Australia are female. You don't think that's true? Ever played Candy Crush or Words With Friends on your phone? What about Angry Birds? If so, then you're a gamer!

But those of us who aren't avid players of games might struggle to understand just why some games are so engaging for young people, so engrossing, so all-consuming.

Take, for example, Minecraft. Why is it that a game that looks so basic has been able to dominate the gaming landscape for so long, particularly given that games look so good right now?

When my son was six, he came to me and said, 'I've built a chest and put my stuff in it, so when I'm exploring for a new village, if a Creeper gets me, at least I won't lose all my stuff.'

If you've never played Minecraft it's likely that this sentence makes little sense. But as someone who has a working knowledge of the game, I have to admit to being proud of the way my son was approaching it. What he was saying in essence was: 'Dad, I've decided to challenge myself, but in doing so I'm well aware of the associated risks and as such I've taken the requisite steps to develop a strategy to deal with failure.'

Games like Minecraft not only capture the imagination of children, they can help teach kids the skills required to be resilient, and much more, and it is important that rather than dismissing such games as a 'waste of time', teachers, parents and maybe even employers understand the mechanics of these games so they can engage the next generation.

Minecraft is something of a sensation. Unless you're a parent, of course, in which case it's most likely the cause of more than a few issues at home. But why is Minecraft so compelling for kids? Actually a better question is, 'Why is Minecraft so *engaging*?'

WHAT IS ENGAGEMENT?

What is engagement and how is it nurtured?

Many educators, parents and students have a varied understanding of what engagement at school looks like.

The Australian *Macquarie Dictionary* defines *engage* as: *verb: 1. To occupy the attention or efforts of (a person etc.)*

Using this definition, it is apparent schools do engage their students. Producing occupied and busy students appears to be the goal that many schools strive for, and regularly achieve.

Think about your kids' crammed academic curriculum, extracurricular clubs and homework schedules. Think about how much time their school demands, and how their involvement is then rewarded via awards, badges, report comments, assembly appearances or grades.

In schools, compliance is sometimes regarded as engagement. 'Does he follow the rules? Does she sit quietly in class, raise her hand to speak and wear her uniform correctly?' We'll describe a student as engaged if they do no more than conform to what is expected.

While the compliant student may still do well in school, by mistaking conformity and compliance for engagement, we miss out on the real benefits of genuine engagement.

The *Macquarie Dictionary* offers another definition that I'd like to explore further: *Engage – verb: 3. To attract and hold fast: to engage the attention: to engage someone's interest.*

This got me thinking. Do we attract students to learning? Or push them into it?

By exploring the literature around engagement, we find it is defined in many ways, but generally these definitions share common ground, and that is: *The sense of living a life high on interest, curiosity and absorption. Engaged individuals pursue goals with determination and vitality.*

Research has shown that adolescents who had a sense of engagement reported higher levels of wellbeing, life satisfaction and less problematic social behaviours.[2] And to help us convince those colleagues of ours who believe school is only about test scores: these students also reported higher grades.

So, clearly, engagement is everyone's business. But be honest – are your kids genuinely engaged?

LEVELS OF ENGAGEMENT

Rather than describing students as either engaged or disengaged, we can consider *levels* or a *continuum of engagement*. This is based on the work of Phil Schlechty.[3]

- **Rebellion** – this is the student who refuses to do any work/activity. He disrupts the class and engages in inappropriate behaviour.
- **Retreatism** – this student does everything they can to get out of doing whatever it is they are supposed to be doing. But typically they are not disruptive.
- **Passive compliance** – this student is doing all that is asked of them but they do not understand why.
- **Ritual engagement** – this student knows exactly why she's doing the work in class. Everyone else is. She knows that she needs good grades to get to university, but she doesn't really see the point of what she's learning in the *here and now.*
- **Authentic engagement** – this student associates the work with personal meaning and sees its value.

In a study conducted with schools in low socioeconomic areas, academics from Western Sydney University suggested we move our thinking of engagement from being merely 'on task' to peak engagement being when you are 'in task'.[4]

The notion of being 'in task' is similar to the state that psychologist Mihaly Csikszentmihalyi describes as 'flow', in which one is 'completely involved in an activity for its own sake. The ego falls away. Time flies. Every action, movement and thought follows inevitably from the previous one, like playing jazz. Your whole being is involved, and you're using your skills to the utmost.'[5]

Being in task or in flow is when an hour feels like ten minutes. The opposite is when ten minutes feels – like – an – hour. You can appreciate how it is possible to be in task by being kept busy, and only be passively or ritualistically engaging without ever reaching peak engagement. Concepts like 'flow' and 'in task' help us consider something more.

In order to be in task or achieve a state of flow, scholars argue that intrinsic motivation is essential. If you're not intrinsically motivated, then by definition you are doing something purely for extrinsic purposes: following orders, reward or the avoidance of punishment. Therefore, intrinsic motivation is a prerequisite for authentic engagement.

INTRINSIC MOTIVATION

According to Ryan and Deci, two of the most prominent motivation and wellbeing researchers in the world,[6] for an individual to be intrinsically motivated they need a sense of:

- **Autonomy** – a sense that they have a choice in the what, why, when and how they do something.
- **Competence/Mastery** – they are striving to improve, not just going over old ground, or moving at too slow a pace.
- **Belonging/Purpose** – the sense that what they are doing has a real relevance to them and the world around them.

WHY IS MINECRAFT SO ENGAGING?

It's these insights into self-determination theory and 'flow' that start to explain why Minecraft, despite its rudimentary graphics, is so popular. In an age when graphics are so good, this game still holds sway because of its understanding of the human psyche. Minecraft is nothing like the games we used to play.

To get a better understanding of this, it's worth taking a trip down memory lane. Do you remember playing Pac-Man? Or perhaps you played pinball at the arcade. Pac-Man was essentially the virtual version of pinball – you had to navigate a ball around a maze, avoiding stuff. But consider this: when you loaded up Pac-Man on your Atari, how much *choice* did you have with regard to how you would play? In short: not much. You could go left or right, and then up or down.

You couldn't, for example, choose to be a ghost. You *had* to be Pac-Man. Upon seeing the maze was the same as you'd played hundreds of times before, you couldn't choose to design and build your own.

You couldn't even really play it with two players. You thought you were playing two players, but in reality you were just waiting for your friend to die so you could have a go. There was no collaboration or teamwork; in fact, the better your friends were at the game, the more likely it was that you wouldn't have enjoyed playing Pac-Man, because you never got a go!

And do you remember how many lives we got in Pac-Man? One – two – three. And then what? Game Over. Start again. From the beginning.

So while looking back through rose-tinted glasses, we might think Pac-Man was a great game – and it was for its time – but it's unlikely that it would dominate our thoughts to such an extent that we would drive our parents and teachers crazy about it.

With the arrival of the Sega Mega Drive and the Nintendo 64 consoles, new games were created with characters that endure to this day, with Sonic the Hedgehog, Link and the Super Mario Bros. to name a few. The way in which players could interact with the games and characters continued to develop also, from two players only being able to play on the same platform either following, or restricted by, each other's movements, to what is now known as split-screen, where players can move around worlds independently.

The shift in the way people have played games on consoles has been fuelled by the development of gaming consoles like Sony's PlayStation, Microsoft's Xbox and, perhaps to a lesser extent, Nintendo's Wii console. For the purpose of this illustration, let's follow the development of the market leader, the Sony PlayStation.

In 1994, Sony released its first PlayStation in Japan. Releases followed in other countries a year later. By 1998, Sony had sold 50 million units. The top-selling game was a racing car game called Gran Turismo. Its popularity was largely due to the incredibly realistic graphics and game play. By the turn of the century, the PlayStation would go on to become the first console to sell 100 million units worldwide.

The benchmark had been set, and to follow that up Sony knew they had to do something special. In 2000 they released the PlayStation 2. The 'something special' was the ability to play online.

Not only were gamers able to play split-screen with their friends in realistic settings, they were now able to play with or against pretty much anyone, anywhere, anytime. The biggest-selling game on the PlayStation 2 was the somewhat controversial Grand Theft Auto.

The PlayStation 3 arrived to much fanfare, with a significant increase in processing power, the ability to play games that not only looked amazing but were seemingly infinite, as well as the ability to opt in or out of various aspects of the game. In short, gamers were offered a narrative for the game, but could take on various – often different – challenges to the ones their friends might choose. It was like a twenty-first-century version of 'Choose Your Own Adventure' books. The realistic graphics, along with more ownership of how to play and the increasing online options for gameplay, meant that the most popular games on the PlayStation 3 were – again – Grand Theft Auto and the Call of Duty warfare games.

So given gamers' desire for better-looking games, and apparently blood and gore, how could it be that at a time when the PlayStation 4 was released, and games have never looked better, a game that looks like Minecraft – with not a drop of blood or hint of criminal behaviour to be found – became one of the most played and talked-about games in the world? In 2014 Microsoft saw fit to buy the game for 2.5 billion US dollars, a move that looks to have been a smart one given that in 2016 – on average, across all devices – 53 000 people bought the game *every day*.

Why? How can this be? It. Looks. Rubbish.

It turns out that Minecraft does something that most other games don't. For the past twenty years, game designers had effectively been saying, 'Here's an even better-looking version of this game, go play it.' Minecraft came along and said, 'Here's a space, what do you want to do in it?'

Minecraft is what is called a 'sandbox' game, in which there are very few limitations placed on the gamer. Players can roam, interact with and change the virtual world at will.

The autonomy afforded to gamers in sandbox games like Minecraft is hard to fathom when compared with our experiences of playing games like Pac-Man or Sonic the Hedgehog. The manner in which gamers can approach and interact, even change the game is completely different to gamers of yesteryear.

Gamers literally create their own worlds, in which they can do almost whatever they want. They can build, make games of their own and collaborate in online spaces on projects as diverse as creating scale replicas of cities around the world, to showing examples of art in a global art gallery built inside of Minecraft.[7] Gamers are also able to create their own modifications or 'mods' that other gamers can download. These mods enable players to change the dynamics of the game almost in their entirety.

WHY DON'T KIDS GIVE UP ON GAMES?

The ability to 'choose your own adventure' has engaged young and old alike for years, but why is it kids will fail over and over at a video game and keep coming back for more, but only need to fail two or three times in class and give up?

When I pose this question to teachers or parents, I'm often met with responses like, 'There's anonymity online, it's low stakes, it's just a game', or "Cos games are fun! D'oh!'

In my mind this implies that adults really do not understand the gaming world. Anonymity may be a factor for some but, to be clear, some of your kids will be better known online – on the other side of the world – than perhaps they are on the other side of their school playground. And I'm not talking in some kind of scary online predator way, I'm talking about young people known though their gamer-tags (unique player identification – mine, for example, is Hazla77) and because of their exploits in online worlds or competitions.

And do you really think games are fun? Have you ever watched a kid playing a video game? Look at their face: you'll see determination, often anger or disappointment. It's not all laughs and giggles. But this offers an insight into the human psyche. It turns out that humans like to struggle with things, as long as they can see the pathway to improvement. It's a concept the late Seymour Papert called 'Hard

Fun'. Kids rarely play games that they master easily because that's boring.

Game designers have known this years, that's why levels of games have always got increasingly difficult – from Space Invaders through to Angry Birds, game designers know they need to have gamers in what I call the 'Stretch Zone', but academics might refer to Vygotsky's Zone of Proximal Development. If you remember the concept of flow from earlier, they share many similarities.

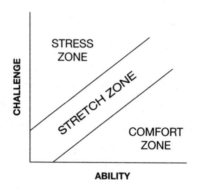

Consider Angry Birds. If you haven't played it, download it now to your phone. It's free. Level one starts off with a simple proposition. After demonstrating how to move the birds using your finger on the screen, you have three attempts to knock the building down and 'kill' the sole green pig, using the red birds.

It usually only takes a few attempts before you've achieved your objective, and you're on to Level 2. Level 2 adds a slight variation and complexity, but not enough to suggest to the gamer it's impossible. By Level 23, the variations and complexities are vast, with multiple pigs hiding in weird and wonderful locations, with additional 'breeds' of birds at your disposal, all with differing dynamics.

If Angry Birds only stayed on or around Level 1, you'd get into and stay in your Comfort Zone. If the game started on Level 23, many would be in their Stress Zone. Game designers recognise that if players stay too long in either of these zones, they stop playing. An incremental rise in difficulty ensures that players are constantly in their Stretch Zone.

And yes, Pac-Man did this, that's why it was fun for us, and this style of game continues to be popular – particularly with older generations. But it's this layer of mastery combined with the autonomy that sandbox games like Minecraft afford that is the secret. It's this combination that encourages players to exhibit behaviours that are actually beneficial in learning, and maybe even life.

I realise that might be pushing it a little, but bear with me as we head off on another tangent and talk about mindset and how it might impact your ability to learn, grow and develop.

WHAT IS MINDSET?

Carol Dweck, PhD from Stanford University, asserts that our mindset, either fixed or growth, can determine our ability to develop new skills and improve existing ones. Since Dweck's book *Mindset – The New Psychology of Success* has been published, many in educational circles have started exploring the concepts of fixed and growth mindsets. First of all, let's look at the fixed mindset.

In a fixed mindset, individuals believe that their abilities and the talents of those around them are predetermined, and a result of genetics. Perhaps they believe that they're 'not a maths person' or they 'don't have a creative bone in their body'. And, to compound that belief, they are of the opinion that no amount of effort can change that.

Perhaps surprisingly, some students who do well at school can also be stuck in a fixed mindset. These students have been told they are really smart, a natural in a certain subject or particularly talented. When they come up against a challenge, as they will invariably do, they feel as though they might not be as smart as people say, otherwise it wouldn't be such a struggle. Dweck's research shows that these students would rather disengage from learning than get less-than-perfect scores. They'd rather lie about a performance in an exam than admit they only scored 15/20.

Unfortunately, some of what we do in schools only serves to reinforce this mindset. Grading, streaming, Gifted & Talented classes, etc. – if not handled properly – can all have negative effects not only on the kids who don't do well in school but also on those who, to all intents and purposes, appear to be successful. In schools, a fixed mindset in students can lead them to believing either that they don't *need to* learn any more or that they *can't* learn any more. Both are dangerous opinions to hold in environments that are all about learning!

However, those in a growth mindset understand that regardless of their abilities and talents, they – whether they are superstars or struggling – have the potential to improve, do things differently and see the benefit of sharing their experiences and time.

In a growth mindset, individuals are concerned with improvement for improvement's sake. Not for the sake of recognition. They take on feedback in a constructive fashion as opposed to seeing it as criticism. Growth mindsets also enable us to recognise and celebrate the successes of others rather than feel threatened by them. And, importantly, those with a growth mindset actively seek out challenges rather than expend their energy trying to avoid them.

Dweck argues that our mindsets are often a product of our environment. How does your environment encourage growth mindsets in your community? Or does it perpetuate a stereotype along the lines of 'Kids from round here don't go to uni', or 'He'll struggle, coming from that family'?

I have long argued that a growth mindset – a belief that we can improve our abilities and talents through effort and effective feedback – should be the number one 'tool' we give to our students. Obviously, this is easier said than done but there are some strategies schools can employ to encourage the development of a growth mindset. Dweck argues that we should praise effort as opposed to outcomes, and be as specific as possible with regard to what we're praising. For example, instead of saying, 'Well done, you didn't make any mistakes', which can be interpreted as meaning mistakes are to be avoided at all costs, we could say, 'Well done. You did such careful work, and really paid attention, that's why you didn't make any silly mistakes.' There is a subtle but very important difference between these two pieces of feedback.

I am constantly urging parents to stop asking their children, 'What did you get?' and start asking, 'What did you get out of it?' And to please stop asking what other kids in the class got. Really that is not the most important question after asking how your child performed.

How does Minecraft develop a growth mindset?

Bring it back to Minecraft. Consider the behaviours that Dweck suggests are representative of having a growth mindset:

- Seeking out and embracing challenge.
- Persisting in the face of setbacks.
- Revelling in the struggle and the need for effort.
- Learning from feedback and critique.
- Being inspired by the success of others.

Minecraft encourages every one of these behaviours. It encourages adopting a growth mindset towards mastery. Players in Minecraft have ownership of their progress. What I mean by that is, because of the constant feedback loops in games, they can articulate where the player has been successful and where potential issues might arise. When they suffer a setback in the game, they are usually able to tell you why they've experienced such a setback and how they might go about addressing it in future attempts. And, crucially, they get to have another go immediately.

Just for a second, compare this to school. Students often don't know if they're on the right track, that's why they have to ask, 'Miss, is this right?' They often don't know where they went wrong, that's why they ask, 'Sir, what did I lose marks for?' And they rarely act on the feedback they get, as research shows that students who get high marks feel they don't need to read the comments, and those who get low marks don't want to. Besides, students are rarely able to resubmit their work anyway, because the class has moved on to a new topic.

But without the final ingredient of self-determination theory, Minecraft wouldn't be the phenomenon that it is. And that ingredient is purpose. Players can determine their own purpose for playing.

The autonomy afforded the player means you could take ten players and find each to be playing Minecraft with ten different purposes. In this sense, Minecraft is truly personalised. Yet it hasn't been personalised for the players by the game designer; rather, the designer has created a space where players can determine their own purpose.

This is why Minecraft is truly engaging and why, as adults, whether you are parents, teachers or employers, you would do well to recognise the mechanics behind it.

I'm not saying that the way to engage young people is to play Minecraft, I'm saying explore how you can create an environment – home, school or workplace – that encourages individual autonomy and a mastery or growth mindset, and allows for a wider discussion about the purpose of what we do, so young people (and everyone else for that matter) can find *their* reason for engaging.

And maybe, just maybe, this might be a more proactive way of getting kids off their screens than merely banning them.

WHAT CAN TEACHERS DO?

- Reduce the amount of grading, at least publicly.
- Use formative assessment strategies to give students more 'ownership' of their learning.
- Think about engagement as being 'in task' rather than 'on task'.
- Think about engagement 'beyond' the classroom through innovative extracurricular offerings and service learning.

WHAT CAN PARENTS DO?

- Recognise that you're not as illiterate as you think, you're probably 'gaming' more than you realise.
- Play games with your kids.
- Give kids 'real world' opportunities to experience autonomy, mastery and purpose by:
  1. Not overscheduling their extracurricular activities. It's hard to have autonomy if you have no time.
  2. Place less emphasis on the outcomes and more on the process.

Author biography

Dan Haesler works with organisations around issues of engagement, wellbeing, mindset and leadership. As well as schools, he has consulted to government education projects, corporate business, The Black Dog Institute and other not-for-profit organisations. Dan is an international keynote speaker, regularly features in the media, and writes a monthly column in the *Australian Teacher Magazine*. Dan's first book, *#SchoolOfThought*, is now available on his website and all profits will go to supporting the Indigenous Literacy Foundation.

www.danhaesler.com

See also:

Chapter 18. What is Resilience and How to Do It
Chapter 20: Using Positive Psychology
Chapter 21: Food, Mood and Mental Health
Chapter 22: Understanding the Teenage Brain

Further reading:

Dweck, Carol 2012, *Mindset*, Little, Brown, London.
Pink, DH 2004, *Drive*, Penguin Putnam Inc, New York.

 For more online resources visit:
generationnext.com.au/handbook

20. USING POSITIVE PSYCHOLOGY

Dr Justin Coulson

Positive Psychology offers evidence-based strategies to support simple interventions to elevate wellbeing and resilience in our teens.

INTRODUCTION

As a child, at what age were you the happiest? When were you the most hopeful about the future? When did you feel like the world made the most sense and you were safest?

Some years ago a major corporation asked me to review the literature on children's wellbeing. They were interested in the age of greatest happiness for children. While individual, family and community factors all play significant parts in the extent to which a child experiences heightened wellbeing, data from around the world pointed to a couple of central findings:

1. Children below around age seven or eight are probably too young to tell us how happy they are. They're not really thinking about it.
2. Once they do start thinking it through, age eight seems to be the age at which they rate their happiness as highest.
3. From the age of eight, there is a general downward trajectory of happiness – as well as hope, resilience and wellbeing – bottoming out around the age of sixteen to seventeen years.

Indeed, it seems that happiness and wellbeing (which are different things) seem to be unsatisfyingly low by the time our children are ensconced in adolescence.

Resilient Youth is a not-for-profit group run by highly regarded Australian child and adolescent psychologist Andrew Fuller. The organisation has collected resilience data from 160 000 Australian children in over 600 communities throughout the country. The data highlights this pattern of wellbeing and resilience occurring in Australia in the same way it has in the United Kingdom and the USA. From Years Three to Twelve, 43 per cent of students (47 per cent of girls and 40 per cent of boys) have good or high levels of resilience. In other words, a little under half of our children aged eight to eighteen are in relatively good shape.

This is a wide age range, though. Our children experience significant developmental changes from ages eight (Year Three) through to eighteen (Year Twelve or equivalent). Think of a young Year Three child and consider the tremendous development that needs to occur for her to become a high school graduate and young adult in a decade's time. So many things will impact on her resilience and wellbeing: physical changes, neurological development, social growth and learning, academic pressures, identity, character and personality development will affect her happiness, life satisfaction and wellbeing across this age span. So, too, will the various life experiences that this girl will encounter – in her family, at school, with her friends and in a range of other settings that can help or hinder her resilience and wellbeing for her entire life.

When we examine Resilient Youth's data by age, we see a distinct pattern emerging. The results show a steady drop from 59 per cent of students reporting good or high levels of resilience in primary school to 27 per cent by Years Eleven and Twelve. As my previous research pointed out, children are still doing best around the age of eight, and are most likely to be struggling around age seventeen, regardless of the wellbeing indices.

Positive Psychology offers evidence-based strategies to turn this wellbeing deficit around. While it cannot be a silver bullet – and arguably nothing can – there is strong science supporting simple interventions to elevate wellbeing and resilience in our teens.

In this chapter I'll explore just three of those ideas: using strengths, growing gratitude and building hope. I'll provide some simple science that underpins the ideas, share real stories that show how these interventions can impact individual lives for the better, and offer a handful of pointers to help you start implementing them.

STRENGTHS AND ADOLESCENT WELLBEING

Mandy was organising a 'night of excellence' for the girls aged twelve to seventeen in her local church group. This was to be a celebration to wind up the year. But as Mandy considered her plans for the event, she realised that the night of excellence might be a night of humiliation for some of the girls. 'We're supposed to be recognising the achievements and milestones that each of the girls has reached this year. But some of them are struggling. Some of them haven't really achieved anything to speak of. And if we were to acknowledge some of their "achievements" it would seem tokenistic, particularly when they're being compared to the other girls' achievements.

'We have girls who are from families where they have lots of resources, and so they receive lots of opportunities. And we have girls from families where they are really struggling, and so they don't really receive any opportunities. And if we want to acknowledge every girl so no one is left out, some of the awards and recognition will look really slack. Are we better to acknowledge minor accomplishments and stuff that's not really that excellent? Or should we leave out the girls who don't really have much to show for the year?'

My suggestion was a simple one, and I had no idea if it might work. 'Why don't you invite each of the girls' mums to prepare a two- or three-minute talk, detailing their daughter's character strengths? Instead of focusing on their external achievements, shift the focus to internal growth and character.'

The idea was novel, but Mandy liked it. Several weeks later I heard back from her.

I listened intently as she described the beautiful, kind things that the mothers had said about their daughters the previous night. She described the tremendous outpouring of emotions that everyone had experienced as mothers spoke of the remarkable strengths, attributes and character their daughters possessed. Several boxes of tissues had been required, and a feeling of psychological and emotional safety had encompassed all who attended.

Mandy continued: 'Something even more incredible happened today though.' Her voice caught. Then came the tears, flowing freely as she told me of a phone call she had received from an overwhelmed and profoundly grateful mother who had attended the evening. 'Nikki is a mum who has it all together. She has a master's degree, the big house, the wealthy husband who loves her like mad. She has the perfect, happy family. She's got the whole package. This morning she called me to say thanks for last night. Nikki's fourteen-year-old daughter, Penelope, was really emotional when her mum shared her thoughts. Like, almost out-of-control emotional.'

Mandy explained that the tears had turned into uncontrollable heaving sobs and Penelope had to leave the room to compose herself. By the end of the evening Penelope had calmed down, but she was still weeping openly and clinging to her mother's side. 'When they got home,' Mandy continued, 'Nikki sat with Penelope on the couch while she cried. After a while she finally said, "What is going on with you? I've never seen you cry like this. Is everything okay? Did I say something wrong?"

'Penelope let go of her mum and asked, "Mum, do you really believe those things that you said about me tonight?"

'"Of course I do, sweetheart. I would never say it if I didn't mean it. Why do you ask?"

'"I've never heard you say anything like that to me before. I just thought you always saw me as a nuisance."'

Mandy described how overwhelmed Nikki and her daughter were, and how the experience had drawn them closer together. Through the experience, Penelope had an opportunity to see herself differently, recognise her strengths and use them as resources to build her resilience.

What are strengths?

How would you define a strength? We use the term all the time, but what does it mean?

Character strengths refer to the virtues and abilities a person possesses that help him or her become a better person. My favourite definition of a strength is that it is a 'potential for excellence' that is inside each of us. Strengths are cultivated through:

- developing an awareness they exist;
- finding ways to access them; and
- making the effort to both expand them and utilise them every day.

Deep inside each of our children is a remarkable capacity to be excellent in something. Some people call it their 'spark'. This suggests a few important things that we should consider. First, strengths are intrinsic, or authentic, or pre-existing. They're a part of who we are and we just need to tap into them. Strengths allow us to perform at a high and consistent level of competence.

DEFINITION

Strengths are abilities or characteristics that:

- are pre-existing;
- feel authentic;
- energise us;
- we perform at a high level of competence.

But there's more to it than that. We feel *strong* when we use our strengths. They help us to feel energised, positive and passionate. This means it's more than just doing something well. It's doing something that enlivens us, lifts us up, engages us and makes us feel we are being who we were born to be!

Using signature strengths is one of the most commonly cited Positive Psychology interventions. Two giants of the Positive Psychology world, the late Professor Christopher Peterson and Professor Martin Seligman, developed a classification framework for character strengths and virtues, based on a broad foundation of philosophical (rather than empirical) views of morality, goodness and character. The model describes six virtues – wisdom and knowledge, courage, humanity, justice, temperance and transcendence – that are considered to be universally prized and sought after across both time and culture. These six virtues act as broad umbrella terms for twenty-four character strengths such as creativity, curiosity, love of learning, perseverance, honesty, zest, kindness, social intelligence, fairness, leadership, forgiveness, humour, spirituality and gratitude.

CHARACTER STRENGTHS AND WELLBEING IN ADOLESCENTS

There is only a small body of research that has been conducted on character strengths and teenagers. One of the most substantive studies involved following a cohort of Year Nine students for two years, measuring their wellbeing, strengths and other variables. The sample in this study was from a relatively wealthy, predominantly white, middle-class demographic. The most common strengths among youth aged thirteen to fifteen years were gratitude, humour and love. Prudence, forgiveness, self-regulation and religiosity were the least common strengths in this cohort. There were also some small gender differences in this study, with females demonstrating the strengths of fairness, kindness and perspective to a greater degree than males within their cohort. Reliably, a significant positive linear relationship exists between wellbeing and character strengths. However, those with low and average strengths seem to benefit most from interventions that promote strength development.

Young people displayed strengths of the heart, such as hope, the capacity to love and be loved, gratitude and zest, and these strengths were linked with wellbeing to a greater extent than strengths of the mind (such as curiosity and love of learning). Strengths that connected teens to others appeared particularly important for wellbeing, because relationships are ultimately at the heart of wellbeing. The research showed that strengths dealing with relationship capacity predicted fewer depressive symptoms across the two-year period of their study. Where children were low on 'other-directed' strengths at the start of Year Nine, they were significantly more likely to report increased depressive symptoms by the end of Year Ten. Beyond these 'other-directed' strengths, transcendence strengths such as meaning and purpose were strong predictors of wellbeing. This means that students reporting low levels of transcendent strengths at the commencement of the study experienced lower life satisfaction for the two years of the study than other children. Therefore, not all strengths relate to wellbeing the same way. Social strengths and transcendent strengths are powerful and important predictors of wellbeing – for young people and for adults.

Additionally, other studies in educational settings have shown that using strengths increases intrinsic motivation in students, and students who can use their strengths best are most likely to succeed academically and socially.

Maria Martínez-Martí and Willibald Ruch, two psychology researchers in Switzerland, carried out a study with just over 360 participants. The study showed significant positive correlations between character strengths and resilience. Strengths mattered for the development of resilience over and above variables like income and education. Strengths contributed to wellbeing beyond the contribution of people feeling positive, having self-belief, being optimistic, having good relationships, enjoying high self-esteem and being satisfied with life. Using strengths actually does build resilience.

Think of what this means in regards to the children and adolescents we work with (or are raising). Are they aware of their strengths? Do they have parents who tell them how strong they are – and how they're strong? Or are we like Nikki, failing to identify and encourage our children to use their strengths? Crucially for their resilience, each day at school, what opportunities do they have to use their strengths? For some children it is easy to feel strong at school. These children have remarkable academic aptitude, or resonate with a particular subject. Some children thrive in social situations and school feeds that strength, buoying them through the day. But for others school can be a place that suffocates strengths. They may have strengths in domains outside of the typical structures that schools create and demand conformity to. They may be creatives, or energisers. Perhaps they prefer manual manipulation of matter, or have exceptional mechanical aptitude or athletic strength, but the school day offers (in some cases) little to enhance those strengths.

HERE ARE SOME SIMPLE IDEAS TO DISCOVER STRENGTHS

- Show pictures of various pop-culture icons, cartoon characters or other famous-ish people and have your children identify their strengths. Do the same with characters in books you read to (or with) them.
- Get children to identify the strengths of parents or friends (but be warned that this can backfire with witty adolescents).
- Find private and sincere ways to emphasise your child's/ student's strengths (positive psychologists call this strength-spotting) and invite them to find opportunities to use them more each day.

Using strengths daily – particularly in the service of others – builds wellbeing, increases engagement, improves productivity and makes people more resilient. But we need a clear language around strengths. Our young people need to know what they are, be able to identify them and work out how to use them in order to get the benefits. Practise spotting strengths in your family members and give them opportunities to use these strengths, and their resilience will increase.

Of course, school requires our children to demonstrate competencies that are important for getting along in life. But when strengths aren't an integral part of our children's day, is it any wonder that they feel weakened, disengaged, and that their resilience drops? Days become drudgery when we do not use our strengths. When school does not offer the opportunities our children require to develop and utilise their strengths, we can look elsewhere to help bolster and develop our children's strengths. The most obvious option is after-school activities including sport, art, writing, music, languages, drama or community-based opportunities like scouts, guides, cadets or other groups. Participation in these activities will be most helpful when it aligns with children's natural strengths, and when they experience high levels of engagement. Our children will develop competence, which builds confidence. They'll learn to think more flexibly, develop relationships, create a sense of identity and persist in order to develop. And we will be able to learn to be patient and encouraging, and find that balance between pushing our children to continue in an activity when they struggle, and letting them stop because it does not align with their strengths, their values or their passions.

DEVELOPING AN ATTITUDE OF GRATITUDE

Gratitude has been called the 'mother of all virtues' but has received surprisingly little scholarly attention. Despite this, gratitude has become the flagship construct of Positive Psychology.

Gratitude can be described as either a state or a trait. Some people feel grateful in some situations (state), and some people seem grateful all the time (trait). In either case, gratitude is a two-part process requiring:

1. recognition of something good in life, and then
2. acknowledgement of that goodness, either to the self or to the source of that goodness.

Those with the trait of gratitude possess a pervasive orientation towards noticing and expressing appreciation, whether for positive or negative circumstances. Indeed, many trials, difficulties and challenges can be catalysts for expressions of gratitude through meaning extracted from experience. If you have ever been through a tough time and looked back at that experience with appreciation for the growth or learning it offered you, then you have experienced the 'benefit-finding' aspects of gratitude for negative experiences.

As an emotion, gratitude focuses the individual on what is positive in his or her world, irrespective of the source, and creates a feeling of appreciation. This feeling orients the individual towards prosocial and positive cognitions and behaviours.

Gratitude is positively related to, or has positive effects upon, all wellbeing indicators. This may, in part, be due to the positive relationship gratitude has with personality characteristics such as emotional warmth, gregariousness, activity seeking, trust, altruism and tender-mindedness. Grateful people appear to be more socially capable and more open to ideas. They also sleep better and enjoy better health. Considering these correlates, it is not surprising to find that the more grateful people are, the better they perceive their relationships to be, the more they show a willingness to forgive, the more they feel peer and family support as adolescents, and the stronger they see their relationships. One study even showed that gratitude promotes more effective conflict resolution. Additional experiments have concluded that gratitude also leads to helping behaviour. And grateful people experience higher levels of wellbeing than those who are less grateful. These are the kinds of things that make adolescents happier and more resilient.

Gratitude is negatively related to hostility and anger, and emotional vulnerability. Gratitude has also been inversely linked with feeling negative and experiencing stress.

But are our young people grateful? Or entitled? As long ago as the 1950s, researchers were suggesting that children are not born with gratitude but, rather, that gratitude is a learned virtue that must be developed. While young children know to be thankful for gifts from an early age, the world's most prominent gratitude researchers today argue that a more authentic (but still formative) gratitude develops from the ages of seven to ten years.

Due to the cognitive complexity of gratitude, adolescence may be a particularly effective time to introduce gratitude as a habit that can foster wellbeing. By this point in their lives, most children are likely to have the capacity to recognise the contribution of others in their lives, and have the ability to acknowledge it. Studies show that the wellbeing effects are undeniably pronounced for grateful teens. As an example, grateful adolescents are more likely to be involved and absorbed in activities than their more materialistic (and less grateful) peers. Jeff Froh and his colleagues theorised that as adolescents express their gratitude for help received, they may even experience enhanced self-respect.

Some specific research findings of interest include a study of 1035 youth aged fifteen to nineteen years, where students who were more grateful also achieved higher marks at school and better social integration, were more absorbed in activities, had higher life satisfaction and were less envious and depressed. In a study of 221 sixth-grade children, participants were divided into a control group, a gratitude group and a daily hassles group. The gratitude group wrote a daily list of five things for which they were grateful, while their daily hassles counterparts wrote of five hassles from their day. Relative to both the control group and the daily hassles group, the gratitude group were significantly more satisfied with school at the completion of the intervention and then again at a three-week follow-up. This is significant in that a large number of students are dissatisfied with school. Yet students who participated in gratitude exercises were glad to be at school, enjoyed it, found it interesting and enjoyed learning. Two weeks of 'counting blessings' appeared to contribute to positive outcomes at school.

Jeff Froh's studies pointed to something else important: youth who were low in positive emotion (more accurately termed 'affect') experienced significant increases in wellbeing after a gratitude visit (where they wrote a heartfelt letter of thanks to someone and then visited them to read the letter aloud). This wellbeing increase was retained for at least two months. The individual's trait gratitude also increased over this time period. This study emphasised that gratitude may or may not be useful in increasing wellbeing, depending on the level of positive affect the individual possesses. If positive affect is low, then gratitude is significantly beneficial to teenagers.

HERE ARE SOME SIMPLE GRATITUDE INTERVENTIONS THAT CAN BE USEFUL IN FAMILY, CLASSROOM, OR OTHER CONTEXTS

Grateful chatter – look for opportunities to encourage people to share a couple of things they're grateful for.

Grateful writing – in a classroom setting, perhaps an assignment might be to find the beauty in a challenge/adversity, or in nature, or at home, and write about it.

Gratitude walls – in some classrooms, staffrooms and living rooms, parents and teachers have set up a gratitude wall. Those in the family or class or office write down various things they're grateful for and stick them on the wall.

Gratitude letters – writing a gratitude letter is a well-documented, empirically validated way of building relationships through expressions of appreciation. Think of someone who has done something for you that is significant, but who you may never have truly thanked. They may or may not be a family member. Write them a letter detailing everything you can about what they have done and how it has affected you. When the letter is written, take it to the person, read it to them and leave it with them.

Model it – just say thanks.

Tell stories that promote gratitude – children love stories, and stories of gratitude typically elevate wellbeing.

Look for the good – sometimes bad things happen. We experience trials and difficulties. Next time there are struggles, wait for the appropriate time and ask the child what good has come out of that struggle, or what good will come out of it. Benefit-finding is a remarkable way of reconstructing challenges and viewing them as blessings, and is also a strategy for increasing wellbeing. After particularly difficult experiences, gratitude can foster post-traumatic growth (rather than its negative corollary, post-traumatic stress).

It has been said that grateful people don't have what they want – they want what they have. While it is tempting to accuse the upcoming generation of narcissism and entitlement, the evidence doesn't support that position. Young people are grateful. We just need to help them remember by guiding them to gratitude, and encouraging them to express it. As they do, they see that the world really is a wonderful place, and their wellbeing and resilience can improve.

BUILDING HOPE IN ADOLESCENTS

One of my favourite stories describes Christmas morning in the home of two young brothers, aged five and eight. The older brother, who was somewhat pessimistic, was told that he had been very, very good throughout the year, so he should expect something nice from Santa. On Christmas morning he opened his stocking after some coaxing from his parents. Inside he found a beautiful gold watch. He held it carefully, told his parents he appreciated it, and then described all the ways he was worried it might break. There was no excitement; only pessimistic concern for what might happen to the watch in the future.

His younger brother was a vibrant, wide-eyed optimist who was forever getting into trouble. He had been warned that Santa might not visit him because he had not been quite so good as his well-behaved, cautious brother. In spite of the warnings, as soon as he was allowed to, he raced to his stocking and hefted it. There was something in there. He yelped in excited anticipation. He tipped the stocking upside down and jumped backwards as horse droppings fell from the stocking and landed at his feet. In an instant he was racing for the back door. His father called him back and asked him where he thought he was going. The boy responded with excitement, 'Santa brought me a pony but it looks like he's gotten away. I've got to run and find him!'

Understanding optimism and hope

Optimism means we feel good about the future. We are hopeful about it and we expect good things will come, even during – and sometimes because of – the difficulties we face. The optimist is the 'glass-half-full' kind of person. Poets and novelists have written countless odes to optimism, promising rising suns, bright futures and endless possibilities to those with courage, optimism and vision. Optimism is positively related to our psychological wellbeing and physical health.

To better understand optimism, it can be helpful to take a look at its opposite. Pessimism is associated with depression, stress and anxiety. People who are strongly pessimistic expect lousy things to happen in the future, and in some cases develop what we know of as helplessness, believing that when something difficult occurs, nothing they do can make things better, so it's not worth trying anyway.

What about hope? In scientific literature there are some technicalities that distinguish optimism from hope, and they are important. While most of us have a natural tendency towards optimism, it is something of a personality characteristic. Hope, however, is different. Hope can be learned. And while optimism builds wellbeing, hope can be even more powerful. To have hope, we (and our children) need three things:

1. a vision or goal;
2. pathways towards that goal; and
3. something psychologists call agency, or efficacy, which is a belief that by taking action we can achieve our goal.

In a sense, this chapter is an exercise in building hope. It's about giving you a vision, mapping out a strategy and helping you find the belief that you can achieve.

The research on hope is compelling. Hopeful people enjoy more success in life than those without hope. They make more effort. They work towards achieving great things. And whether they actually get to where they hoped to get or not, they often come closer to it than they would have if they had not hoped at all.

How to enhance optimism and create hope

In *The Optimistic Child* Martin Seligman describes a simple conversation that he asks parents to enjoy with their children to encourage a positive future-orientation – or optimism. He suggests tucking our children into bed at night, sitting with them and asking them to describe something that they're looking forward to. Our children will share their hopes and dreams with us. We will learn what is meaningful to them. Trust in our relationships will deepen, and security will be strengthened.

We don't need to be parents or tuck children into bed to have this conversation. What matters is that we give youth the chance to chat about these ideas. This optimistic view of the future is the beginning of true hopefulness.

To generate a more powerful sense of hope, we can work towards meaningful goals with children or students. Take a moment now to reflect on the last meaningful goal you achieved with a student or your own family. What was the goal? How did you plan on getting there? How did you create the belief you could achieve it? How did it feel for you to progress in the right direction? What are you and the children or students you work with aiming for now?

TRY THESE IDEAS TO BUILD HOPE AT HOME OR WITH THE YOUNG PEOPLE YOU WORK WITH

1. Build a future focus: speak to your children about their possible futures. What do they want to achieve and why? Have them imagine their potential best selves. Talk to them about what they're looking forward to. Ask them what they want to have, do and be.

2. Work with them on plans (or pathways): when a child says, 'I want to be a marine biologist', be encouraging and then ask them, 'What do you need to do to get there?' Discuss pathways, options and possibilities. Thinking about the future and making plans is central in fostering hope.

3. When they're stuck, rather than giving them an answer, ask them, 'What do you think is the next best thing to do?' or 'When have you overcome something like this before?' These types of questions promote a sense of agency or efficacy. Rather than having our children rely on us for all of the answers, they can rely on themselves, their resourcefulness and their initiative. They can recall times they've succeeded before and use that to build hope that they can succeed again.

There is nothing more valuable in inoculating young people against depression, anxiety and hopelessness than encouraging hope. Helping them see that there is something to look forward to may be the single most important thing we do each day.

When a science class was struggling one day, a Year Nine teacher stopped the class and wrote on the board, 'THERE IS LIFE AFTER HIGH SCHOOL'. Then the class talked a little about their hopes and dreams. More than a decade later, at the Year Twelve ten-year reunion, students reminded the teacher of that lesson and assured her it was 'the thing' that helped them through high school. Hope is powerful.

There are dozens of ways that we can approach wellbeing with children and students. Some things will resonate for you – or for them – more than others. Having someone by their side who really cares, and who helps them to use their strengths, find the good in their lives and look forward to the future can be all it takes to help them move towards greater resilience and wellbeing.

Author biography

Dr Justin Coulson is one of Australia's most respected relationships speakers, authors, and researchers. He is an Honorary Fellow at the Centre for Positive Psychology at the University of Melbourne's Graduate School of Education, and a Senior Associate at the Positive Psychology Institute. He has authored multiple peer-reviewed journal articles and book chapters, and written a number of popular books and e-books about parenting and happiness. In addition, Dr Coulson writes a weekly parenting advice column for Sydney's *Daily Telegraph*, appears regularly on the *TODAY* show and is the parenting expert at kidspot.com.au – Australia's number one parenting website.

www.happyfamilies.com.au

See also:

Chapter 18: What is Resilience and How to Do It

Chapter 19: Harnessing the Minecraft Mindset for Success

Chapter 21: Food, Mood and Mental Health

Chapter 22: Understanding the Teenage Brain

Further reading:

Deci, EL & Ryan, RM 2000, 'The "what" and "why" of goal pursuits: Human needs and the self-determination of behaviour', *Psychological Inquiry*, vol. 11, pp 227–268.

Fredrickson, BL 2006, *The Broaden-and-Build Theory of Positive Emotions*, Oxford University Press, New York.

Linley, A 2008, *Average to A+: Realising strengths in yourself and others*, CAPP Press, London.

Lopez, SJ & Snyder, CR (Eds), *Oxford Handbook of Positive Psychology* (2nd ed), Oxford University Press, New York, pp 667–677.

Peterson, C & Seligman, MEP 2004, *Character strengths and virtues: A handbook and classification*, Oxford University Press, New York.

Seligman, MEP & Csikszentmihalyi, M 2000, 'Positive psychology: An introduction', *American Psychologist*, vol. 55, pp 5–14.

Seligman, MEP, Ernst, RM, Gillham, J, Reivich, K & Linkins, M 2009, 'Positive education: Positive psychology and classroom interventions', *Oxford Review of Education*, vol. 35, pp 293–311.

Snyder, CR & Lopez, SJ 2007, *Positive psychology: The scientific and practical explorations of human strengths*, Sage Publications, Thousand Oaks.

For more online resources visit:
generationnext.com.au/handbook

21. FOOD, MOOD AND MENTAL HEALTH

Felice Jacka

This chapter will provide an overview of the evidence linking diet to mental health, including in young people. It will provide evidence-based suggestions for the prevention and treatment of common mental health problems, such as depression and anxiety.

INTRODUCTION

Previous chapters have provided a detailed insight into depression in young people – how common it is, its diagnosis and impact, and some of the risk factors and potential solutions. In this chapter we will focus on a particular risk factor for common mental health problems that has only recently come to light: diet.

Over recent decades, the health of the world's population has suffered a major setback due to profound changes in eating habits across countries, cultures and age groups. Sometime back in the twentieth century, big business started to understand that it could manufacture 'food products' that were highly attractive to humans. More than that, they realised that these products were very cheap to produce, could stay 'fresh' for very long periods of time, and were very easy to sell. Indeed, people seemed to almost fall over each other to buy and eat them. As a result, the eating habits of people began to change, first in the west, then across developing countries and traditional cultures. Instead of meat, fish, beans and vegetables as dietary staples, people started eating processed food and drinks, with added sugars, salt, fat, artificial colours and flavours, preservatives, emulsifiers and even artificial sugars. These foods were and are cheap, widely available, socially acceptable and very addictive.

What was the first, most obvious marker of this change in our eating habits? Obesity, of course, along with type 2 diabetes, hypertension and other symptoms of the metabolic syndrome. Now, in 2017, chronic diseases related to poor diet have outstripped infectious diseases, such as HIV and malaria, as the world's greatest killers. Indeed, unhealthy diet is now known to be *the* leading risk factor for early death across the globe. In the USA this year, for the first time, life expectancies actually decreased – mainly as a result of chronic disease related to poor diet.

But there is something extremely important that has not been considered and that is: it's not only our physical health that is affected by these changes to our diets. It's also our mental and brain health.

DIET AND ITS RELATIONSHIP TO MENTAL HEALTH: WHAT DO WE NOW KNOW?

Firstly, it's important to understand that mental disorders, along with drug use and addiction, now account for the leading cause of global disability. They impose a very great burden on individuals, families and communities, and are very expensive to business and the public purse. For this reason, identifying risk factors for mental disorders that are *modifiable* – meaning that we can do something about them – is incredibly important. So many factors that influence the risk for mental health problems, such as genetics or early life stress for example, are very difficult to address. The fact that diet is now known to be a risk factor for depression offers new hope that we can prevent and treat at least some of the burden of depression by dietary strategies.

DIET QUALITY IS CLEARLY RELATED
TO DEPRESSION IN ADULTS

Prior to 2009, there had been a number of studies seeking to examine possible links between the consumption of individual nutrients and foods, and the presence of depression. Many of these studies focused on key nutrients such as folate, other B-group vitamins, and the long chain omega-3 fatty acids that are found predominantly in seafood. An important problem was, of course, that people don't just eat individual nutrients or foods. Thus, medical researchers started to understand that it was more useful to consider the whole of diet, since diet is highly complex in its components, all of which interact in ways that we cannot yet map.

For this reason, the first studies to show that the quality of people's overall diets was related to mental health created a lot of interest. The first of these examined the relationships between dietary patterns and clinical depressive and anxiety disorders in Australian women. This study showed that women whose diets were generally higher in vegetables, fruit, unprocessed beef, lamb, fish and wholegrain foods were less likely to have clinically diagnosed depressive or anxiety disorders, whereas a 'western'-type diet, higher in processed and 'unhealthy' foods, was associated with more depression. In this same group, women with the same healthy dietary pattern were also only half as likely to have bipolar disorder, while those who scored higher on the western dietary pattern and glycaemic load were more likely to have bipolar disorder. Around the same time, two other large studies, from Spain and the UK, showed similar findings. Over the next few years, more and more studies were published, showing the same thing. This was the case across many different countries and cultures. Consistently, no matter what form a 'healthy' diet took – whether it was an Asian one, with fish, seaweed and soy products, or a Mediterranean one, with fish, legumes, nuts, vegetables and olive oil, or even a Scandinavian one, with lots of fish, vegetables and non-processed red meats – people with healthier diets were less likely to have depression and, in many cases, anxiety. Unhealthier diets, which look more similar across the globe (because they come from the same source – big business) were also commonly associated with more depression and anxiety.

Of course, correlation doesn't equal causation. We know that appetite changes are very common in those with depression – some people eat less, while others crave sweet and fatty foods as part of their condition. Also, the links might be explained by other factors that are related to both diet and mental health, such as people's social and financial circumstances, educational levels, age and gender, body weight, and whether they take care of their health in other areas of their lives (exercise, smoking and alcohol consumption). The many studies that examined the associations took pains to consider other such factors that might explain associations between diet and mental health, but these didn't appear to be the reason for the links that were seen. Other studies suggested that diet pre-dated depression. So, the population-based studies were compelling in suggesting that diet was a determinant of mental health in adults. But what about in younger people?

DIET AND ITS RELATIONSHIP TO MENTAL HEALTH IN YOUNG PEOPLE

We know that adolescence is a particularly important period for mental health, with many mental disorders first manifesting in early adolescence. Thus, identifying risk factors that can be *changed* is an especially important task. For this reason, there are now many studies that have also examined the links between diet quality and mental health in young people.

In one of the first studies to examine this question, both a lower intake of healthy foods and an increased intake of unhealthy and processed foods were related to increased depression in more than 7000 young Australian adolescents. In fact, those adolescents in the highest category of 'healthy' diet were only half as likely to be depressed as those in the lowest category, while for those in the highest category of 'unhealthy' diet score, the likelihood of them having depression was increased by nearly 80 per cent. These relationships held true even after taking into account important factors such as their family's socioeconomic status, the educational level of their parents, and levels of family conflict and other such factors in the home. Another Australian study examined approximately 3000 young adolescents and found that diet quality was associated with adolescent mental health over time. In this study, improvements in diet quality over a two-year period were mirrored by improvements in mental health, while reductions in diet quality were associated with worse psychological health.

In common with what is seen in adults, the relationship between diet quality and mental health in adolescents has now been consistently shown in many diverse countries, including China, Germany, Norway and the UK. Once again, the relationships that have been reported seem to be independent of adolescents' family and social environments, their levels of exercise, their weight and their dieting behaviours.

Another important consideration is that of the possible impact of nutrition in very early life and its relationship to the risk of mental health problems in children. Early life experiences and environments have a potent influence on children's behavioural, emotional and learning outcomes, pointing to the central importance of identifying early life risk factors for mental disorders that are modifiable, such as diet, in order to *prevent* mental health problems before they start.

In this context, there is important evidence from a very large Norwegian study of more than 23 000 mothers and their children showing that the children of mothers with unhealthy diets during pregnancy had higher levels of emotional health problems, signified by what are called 'internalising' (crying, sad, anxious) and 'externalising' (angry, tantrum, aggressive) behaviours. The children's diets were also associated with these mental health markers, with both healthy and unhealthy dietary patterns during the first years of life clearly associated with emotional problems in these young children. This study has now received support from two further large studies in the Netherlands and the UK.

IMPROVING DIET TO IMPROVE DEPRESSION: A NEW APPROACH

While the evidence from these large, population-based surveys is very consistent in showing that the quality of people's diets is related to their risk for depression and related disorders across the lifespan, it doesn't answer the question of whether this is a true 'causal' relationship. For this, we need to have intervention studies. These are where we take groups of people and seek to change their diets, looking to see whether such changes have an impact on their symptoms of depression. Such studies are very challenging to do for many reasons. First, to show the prevention of depression, you generally need very large groups of people and to follow them for quite a long time to see who develops depression. Second, getting people to change their diets is notoriously hard. Getting them to report their diets honestly is also difficult. Finally, we can't really put some people into a junk food group as this wouldn't be ethical (this would be a bit like getting some people to smoke and others not to smoke, then following them for years to see who got cancer). However, some very recent and important studies have succeeded and the outcomes of these tell us that there are very exciting possibilities for targeting diet to both prevent and treat depression.

In the PREDIMED study, several thousand older European adults who were deemed to be at increased risk of a heart attack or related event were recruited to take part in the largest dietary intervention study in the world to date. They were randomly assigned to one of three groups and told to follow either the dietary recommendations of the American Heart Association, which focuses on reducing both animal and vegetable fats (the control group), or to one of two groups who were encouraged to change their diet to a Mediterranean-style diet that emphasises the consumption of vegetables, fruit, legumes, fish, olive oil and red wine. One of these groups was also encouraged to substantially increase their consumption of extra virgin olive oil, while the other was encouraged to have at least a handful of raw nuts every day. The participants of this trial were followed for more than two years and the researchers found that those who were in the Mediterranean-type diet groups were less likely to have a heart attack or related event than those in the low-fat control group. But further investigation of the data also showed that those following the Mediterranean-style diet tended to not develop depression either. This was particularly the case for those participants who had the extra nuts as part of their diet. Whether or not nuts hold a particular benefit to mental health has still to be established, but the benefits of a diet high in plant foods, fish and olive oil to both mental and physical health seem pretty clear.

With these findings in mind, a very recent study has now – for the first time – attempted to answer the very important question: 'I'm depressed; if I improve my diet, will it help my depression?'

In the 'Supporting the Modification of lifestyle In Lowered Emotional States' (SMILES) randomised controlled trial, adults with major depressive disorder were recruited and randomly assigned to receive either social support, which is known to be helpful for people with depression, or support from a clinical dietitian, over a three-month period. The dietary group received information and assistance to improve the quality of their current diets, with a focus on increasing the consumption of vegetables, fruits, wholegrains, legumes, fish, lean red meats, olive oil and nuts, while reducing their consumption of unhealthy 'extra' foods, such as sweets, refined cereals, fried food, fast food, processed meats and sugary drinks.

The results of the study, now published in the international journal *BMC Medicine*, showed that participants in the dietary intervention group had a much greater reduction in their depressive symptoms over the three-month period, compared to those in the social support group. At the end of the trial, 32 per cent of those in the dietary support group, compared to 8 per cent of those in the social support group, met criteria for remission of major depression. These results were not explained by changes in physical activity or body weight, but were closely related to the extent of dietary change. Those who adhered more closely to the dietary programme experienced the greatest benefit to their depression symptoms.

These latest findings offer an important new strategy for the treatment of depression. While approximately half of patients with depression are helped by currently available medical and psychological therapies, new treatment options for depression are urgently needed. Importantly, depression also increases the risk of and, in turn, is also increased by common physical illnesses such as obesity, type 2 diabetes and heart disease. Successfully improving the quality of patients' diets should also benefit these illnesses. Thus, this latest study suggests the new possibility of adding clinical dietitians to mental health care teams and making dietitian support available to those experiencing depression.

DIET AND BRAIN HEALTH: COGNITION AND NEURODEVELOPMENT

Finally, there is the very important issue of neurodevelopmental disorders, such as Autism Spectrum Disorders (ASD). The prevalence of these has risen rapidly in the last twenty years or so, although it's an ongoing debate as to whether this reflects an increased recognition and better diagnosis by clinicians, or a true increase. In either case, the evidence that diet in early life (including during gestation) might influence the risk of developmental disorders such as ASD needs to be taken seriously. What we know now is that parents' – both mothers' and fathers' – metabolic health is clearly related to the risk for these disorders in children. In other words, mothers and fathers who are overweight, obese and/or have metabolic disorders such as type 2 diabetes are more likely to have children with ASD or developmental delays. These relationships may be occurring through changes to genetic processes (epigenetics), including those that influence the sperm, through influences on early gut health in children, which is now beginning to be recognised as an important determinant of brain and immune development, or through other pathways – all of which likely interact with each other. The results of these studies are also consistent with what we see in animal experiments where unhealthy diets fed to pregnant animals results in many changes to the brain and behaviour in offspring.

Taken together, these research studies tell us that the changes in dietary habits around the globe are likely to be influencing the prevalence of depression and related mental disorders, and neurodevelopmental disorders. Importantly, they also suggest that the impact of these dietary changes on the global burden of mental disorders is yet to fully appear, given that the harmful changes to food habits are particularly obvious in younger people, who will become parents to the next generation.

WHAT DOES THIS MEAN FOR INDIVIDUALS AND FAMILIES?

What this clearly means is that individuals and families have more reasons than ever to take diet and nutrition seriously. Dietary habits are created early in life and establishing good dietary habits – by setting examples, getting children involved in growing and/or preparing healthy food, and reinforcing the central importance of good nutrition as the essential 'fuel' that powers both physical and mental health – is critical. There are many books and other resources that can help families transition away from a fast food culture to a healthy one. It doesn't need to be expensive – while foods such as fresh fish, organic vegetables and berries are clearly more expensive than many junk foods, there are many studies now to show that a healthy diet can be cheaper than an unhealthy one. Using legumes (such as chickpeas, lentils and beans), brown rice and other whole grains, and even frozen vegetables – which are nutritionally similar to fresh ones – as the basis of meals can allow any family to have a healthy diet on a budget. Making soups and stews with these types of ingredients at the start of the week is also a great idea for time-poor parents. If we want the next generation to have better physical and mental health, to have the best chance at a healthy life and a long lifespan, we owe this to our children and to ourselves.

WHAT DOES THIS MEAN FOR TREATMENT OF MENTAL DISORDERS?

All of this evidence now tells us that diet is likely as important to mental and brain health as it is to physical health. The WHO has long said that 'there is no health without mental health'. We now believe that the opposite is also true and that physical and mental health should be considered two sides of the same coin. In this sense, the same diet and exercise recommendations that are made to prevent and treat common physical illnesses, such as heart disease, are also relevant for mental disorders and brain health. Improving the quality of people's diets would have benefits for the many physical illnesses that commonly accompany depression, such as heart disease, diabetes and obesity. Thus, there is no longer a justification for not addressing the whole person when treating mental illnesses. It may well be that a dietitian will soon become part of every multidisciplinary psychiatric team and that, soon, referrals to dietitians will be common for people with mental disorders.

TAKE-HOME MESSAGES FOR PARENTS

Diet and nutrition are the foundations of physical, mental and brain health for your children *and* the next generation. Don't give up on improving your family's diets – it can take up to six exposures to a new food for kids to accept and eat it. Making healthy food the default in your home, and even learning cooking skills together, will make all the difference to your children's dietary habits over the long term. And it will likely make a big difference to their mental and brain health as well.

TAKE-HOME MESSAGES FOR TEACHERS AND SCHOOL COUNSELLORS/YOUTH WORKERS

Don't ignore the important role of diet in children's mental health and their ability to learn. It is the foundation that allows for learning, positive growth and development. Good nutrition is essential for the brain and without it, teaching and other forms of support are likely to be less effective.

TAKE-HOME MESSAGES FOR PROFESSIONALS

Promoting the importance of healthy diet for mental and brain health does not need a qualification in dietetics or nutrition. Ignore the media messages around gluten-free, paleo, saturated fat vs olive oil, sugar or no sugar: many of these messages are planted by big business and designed to confuse. The message is actually simple and it's this: 'Eat (whole) food, not too much, mostly plants' (Michael Pollan). If there is a suspected food allergy, or the food environment in the home is very poor, provide a referral to a dietitian for expert support.

Author biography

Professor Felice Jacka is an NHMRC Career Development Fellow at Deakin University, where she is Director of the Food and Mood Centre. She is president of the International Society for Nutritional Psychiatry Research (ISNPR) and immediate past president of the Australian Alliance for the Prevention of Mental Disorders (APMD). Professor Jacka has pioneered and led a highly innovative programme of research that examines how individuals' diets, and other lifestyle behaviours, interact with the risk for mental health problems.

www.foodandmoodcentre.com.au

See also:

Chapter 4: Anxiety in Young People
Chapter 5: Depression in Young People
Chapter 18. What is Resilience and How to Do It
Chapter 19: Harnessing the Minecraft Mindset for Success
Chapter 20: Using Positive Psychology
Chapter 22: Understanding the Teenage Brain

Recommended websites:

British Dietetic Association: www.bda.uk.com/foodfacts/home

NHS: www.nhs.uk/Livewell/goodfood

International Society for Nutritional Psychiatry Research: www.ISNPR.org

Drew Ramsey, MD: www.drewramseymd.com

Further reading:

Dawson, SL, Dash, SR & Jacka, FN 2016, 'The Importance of Diet and Gut Health to the Treatment and Prevention of Mental Disorders', *Int Rev Neurobiol*, vol. 131, pp 325–346.

Jacka, FN 2015, 'Lifestyle factors in preventing mental health disorders: An interview with Felice Jacka', *BMC Medicine*, vol. 13(1).

Jacka, FN, Cherbuin, N, Anstey, KJ, Sachdev, P, Butterworth, P 2015, 'Western diet is associated with a smaller hippocampus: A longitudinal investigation', *BMC Medicine*, vol. 13(1).

Jacka, FN, Ystrom, E, Brantsaeter, AL, Karevold, E, Roth, C, Haugen, M, Meltzer, HM, Schjolberg, S & Berk, M 2013, 'Maternal and Early Postnatal Nutrition and Mental Health of Offspring by Age 5 Years: A Prospective Cohort Study', *Journal of the American Academy of Child and Adolescent Psychiatry*, vol. 52(10).

Jacka, FN, Mykletun, A & Berk, M 2012, 'Moving towards a population health approach to primary prevention of common mental disorders', *BMC Medicine*, vol. 10(1).

Jacka, FN, Kremer, PJ, Berk, M, de Silva-Sanigorski, AM, Moodie, M, Leslie, ER, Pasco, JA & Swinburn, BA 2011, 'A Prospective Study of Diet Quality and Mental Health in Adolescents', *PLoS ONE*, vol. 6(9).

Jacka, FN, Pasco, JA, Mykletun, A, Williams, LJ, Hodge, AM, O'Reilly, SL, Nicholson, GC, Kotowicz, MA & Berk, M 2010, 'Association of Western and Traditional Diets With Depression and Anxiety in Women', *American Journal of Psychiatry*, vol. (3).

O'Neil, A, Itsiopoulos, C, Skouteris, H, Opie, RS, Mcphie, S, Hill, B & Jacka, FN 2014, 'Preventing mental health problems in offspring by targeting dietary intake of pregnant women', *BMC Medicine*, vol. 12(208).

Opie, RS, Itsiopoulos, C, Parletta, N, Sanchez-Villegas, A, Akbaraly, T, Ruusunen, A & Jacka, FN 2015, 'Dietary recommendations for the prevention of depression', *Nutritional Neuroscience*.

Sarris, J, Logan, AC, Akbaraly, TN, Amminger, P, Balanzá-Martínez, V, Freeman, MP, Hibbeln, J, Matsuoka, Y, Mischoulon, D, Mizoue, T, Nanri, A, Nishi, D, Ramsey, D, Rucklidge, JJ, Sanchez-Villegas, A, Scholey, A, Su, K-P & Jacka, FN 2015, 'Nutritional medicine as mainstream in psychiatry', *The Lancet Psychiatry*, vol. 2(3).

For more online resources visit:
generationnext.com.au/handbook

22. UNDERSTANDING THE TEENAGE BRAIN

Dr Michael Nagel

Until recently, very little was known about brain development during the teenage years. Advances in research and technology have now provided us with very important insights into the developing teenage brain, which in turn should help us to better understand and engage with young people.

INTRODUCTION

Our understanding of brain development has grown exponentially over the last couple of decades. Neuroscientific research has merged boundaries with many other fields and, as such, the science surrounding the brain and mind is now available to parents and all those who work with and engage young minds every day. In other words, we are gaining far greater access to, and understanding of, the developing brain and there is indeed much attention to be given to the teenage brain. However, in order to better understand the teenage brain and provide a foundation for understanding some of the behaviours associated with being a teenager, a brief introduction to the brain's structures and how it develops is necessary.

THE DEVELOPING BRAIN

The human brain is an amazingly complex, still poorly understood organ. Consisting of various layers and structures, the brain possesses hundreds of billions of cells that bathe one another in chemical messengers that influence moment-to-moment changes of the mind, behaviour and experience. Its complexity is so unmatched by anything in nature that the brain has been described as the most unimaginable thing imaginable, and although we have learned a great deal, most neuroscientists would likely agree that we probably only know about 1 per cent of what we would like to know. What we do know, however, is that the brain starts out as a small collection of cells that becomes a complex super-highway of electro-chemical impulses which shape who we are and what we do.

Chronologically speaking, the brain begins to form about seventeen days after conception. This marks the beginning of an amazing journey of neural development where neurons will generate and migrate to different regions of the brain. Neurons are a type of brain cell that resemble bulbs, with sprouting roots called 'dendrites' and a tail-like structure known as the 'axon'. The dendrites of neurons act like antennae and receive information from other neurons and/or from environmental stimulation. As you read these words right now, your brain is gathering information that passes through your eye to your occipital lobes where it is interpreted and dispersed to other areas of the brain. An important, and sometimes difficult, thing to remember is that seeing isn't happening in your eyes. Nor does hearing take place in your ears or smelling happen in your nose. Your sensory organs take in information, which is translated into electrochemical signals and passed between neurons while your brain decides what to do with the information. This passing of information between neurons occurs across a small gap between axon terminals and dendrites, which is commonly referred to as a 'synapse' and facilitated with the assistance of 'neurotransmitters' (chemical messengers). Everything that you experience is the product of an electrochemical dance that is choreographed for future attention or deemed unimportant and forgotten.

The process of passing information noted above is how the brain 'learns'. When axons send signals that are received by dendrites, via a synapse, learning takes place; and the more that these types of connections are made, the faster and more efficiently the signals move and the more permanent they become. An important aspect of this communication between neurons is that if synapses are used repeatedly, over time they will become 'hardwired' pathways and part of the brain's permanent circuitry. Conversely, if they are not used repeatedly or often enough, they are usually eliminated and much of this occurs during the teenage years. This 'hard-wiring' of pathways appears to be a 'use-it-or-lose-it' process whereby nurture helps to shape nature. In other words, experience plays a pivotal role in 'wiring' the brain. This is perhaps one of the greatest examples of how nature and nurture work together with the end result being the overall development of the mind. Moreover, all human behaviour can be traced to the communication among neurons whereby every thought and experience you have, every emotion you feel, every moment you make and all of your awareness of the world around you is possible because neurons talk to each other. This neural chatter is rampant in the first few years of life and by age three, a child will have more connections in its brain than the paediatrician it visits when unwell. In essence, the brain overcompensates by producing more connections than are needed and then it gets rid of many of those connections during the teenage years. We will revisit that later but at this point it is also significant to note all of this early neural activity leading to a mature brain relies on some important chemicals and for a number of functions to occur over time. The brain does not fully mature until we are in our third decade of life and, as such, full neurodevelopment is actually more marathon than sprint. During this marathon, the teenage years see significant changes to the brain and also the potential for significant behavioural manifestations. There may be some very good reasons why teenagers will do things that leave adults bewildered and those reasons can be found in the changing structures and functions within the teenage brain.

STRUCTURES OF THE BRAIN

The structures of the brain and the maturation of those structures offer important insights into the world of teenagers. The number of structures at play inside anyone's head at any one time are vast in scope and detail and therefore it is prudent to limit this part of the discussion to a broader and perhaps more general perspective of those things going on inside the head of a teenager. In adopting this position, we can start by looking at three regions of prominence within the brain: the brainstem, the limbic system and the cerebrum. It is significant to note that isolating these areas is for descriptive purposes primarily, given that they are intimately connected and work in concert with one another.

The brainstem or region closest to the spine is responsible for functions not under conscious control and where survival responses such as fight or flight are activated. The limbic system or central part of the brain harbours and processes our emotions and memories. Finally, the cerebrum, which contains the occipital, temporal, parietal and frontal lobes, has been recognised as the region where processing environmental stimuli, thinking and consciousness exist. Within the cerebrum, the frontal lobes are integral components of who we are and what we do. In the context of understanding the teenage brain, some very important and relatively new insights have emerged regarding these areas and brain function.

First, there was a time when some believed that many of our cognitive capabilities were mature and readily available on or about the time puberty kicked in. We now know that this is simply a whimsical notion and that the teenage brain undergoes a massive remodelling of many areas that affect everything from logical and responsible thinking to impulse control to sensation seeking and the controlling of one's emotions. Full brain maturation extends beyond the teenage years but there is a lot of work going on between the ears of teenagers. In terms of maturation we know that the survival mechanisms of the brain along with the limbic system or emotional hub of the brain are mature long before the analytical and logical processes of the prefrontal lobes come fully online. This means that teenagers are hot-wired for emotion but often lack the brakes to slow down those emotions when they speed down life's highway of experimentation and experience.

We also know that during the teenage years the brain travels down a pathway of deconstruction whereby it discards unused synaptic connections or prunes away those connections developed in the first three to four years of life as it works towards becoming more efficient. Interestingly, this restructuring occurs in concert with an increase in myelin, or the white matter of the brain. All of these changes are significant and amid all of this restructuring, pruning and growth in myelin, it is important to remember that the brain seems to mature roughly from the bottom up and around to the front, and in different areas and at a different rate for males and females. These changes can have a profound impact on various mechanisms of the mind and on teenage emotions and thought processes, or the lack thereof. The implications of this incredible neural transformation are evident in teenage behaviour and, quite simply, in how teenagers engage in and deal with the world around them. A more detailed look at the changes noted provides us with a great deal of food for thought when it comes to working with and engaging teenage minds. The production of myelin offers a good starting point for such exploration.

MYELIN AND SYNAPTIC PRUNING – THE MATURING BRAIN

Myelin is the white matter of the brain and is actually a fatty material that grows like a sheath around the axons of neurons and acts as an insulator and conductor. Because it acts as an insulator, myelin aids in synaptic communication. Simply stated, more 'myelinated' axons mean a faster and more efficient brain with the end result being that certain activities are easier to learn when regions of the brain are sufficiently myelinated or when our brains become 'fatter'. This is very evident in the early years of a child's life when it is clear that many of a child's capacities do not 'come online' until regions of the brain have received significant myelin growth. For example, vision and motor coordination are very limited at birth because the neural networks responsible for sight and movement aren't working fast enough due to the lack of myelinated axons. Importantly, the last regions of the brain to myelinate completely are the frontal lobes and in particular the prefrontal lobes. This is the region of the brain that considers what is a reasonable response to an adult, what are the implications of getting a piercing and a myriad of other teenage dilemmas.

This process of myelin development noted above is referred to as myelination or myelinisation and is a lengthy journey lasting well into the twenties and resulting in the tripling of the size and weight of the brain. Interestingly, while the teenage brain is expanding its volume of myelin, it is also decreasing its total volume of connections through a process noted earlier as pruning or, more accurately, synaptic pruning.

Synaptic pruning is a vital process with regards to overall brain development. Remember that in the first few years of life, a child's neural connections will come to outnumber those of an adult. On or about the time pubescence begins, and most notably through the teenage years, the brain starts to discard or prune those synaptic regions that are seldom used. This allows the brain to refine itself, become more specialised and more efficient, and process stimulation and information faster. The greatest influence on the connections that the brain maintains and what it decides to discard is found in an individual's own life experiences and environment. Synaptic pruning is an extremely important process of development where the saying 'use it or lose it' attains great implications for teenagers in that the brain is actually being remodelled or reconstructed. Therefore, the experiences that teenagers have – or don't have for that matter – not only impact on teenage emotions, thought processes, learning and behaviour but quite literally shape their brains.

Another important aspect related to the pruning of synapses is that like the production of myelin, the last regions of the brain to be pruned are the prefrontal lobes, or the brain's 'chief executive officer'.

As teenagers engage with the world around them, myelination and pruning are part of a natural developmental stage that can impose on, and give rise to, specific behaviours. Before looking at some of those specific behaviours there is one further aspect of teenage brain development worthy of consideration, namely the influence of certain neurotransmitters.

NEUROTRANSMITTERS AND THE BRAIN

As I mentioned at the beginning of this chapter, neurotransmitters are the chemical messengers released during the communication of information from one neuron to another via synaptic transmissions. The brain produces probably at least fifty, and maybe as many as one hundred, different chemicals that it uses to communicate. During the teenage years some of the important neurotransmitters in our brain seem to have a mind of their own. Three of those that are most pertinent to this discussion on teenagers are melatonin, serotonin and dopamine.

Melatonin is a neurotransmitter that forms part of the system that regulates the sleep–wake cycle associated with our circadian rhythms. This important chemical is produced in the centre of the brain by the pineal gland and when the sun goes down and darkness grows, melatonin levels increase and we feel sleepy. It appears, however, that once puberty kicks in, the release of melatonin declines and seems to be pushed back a couple of hours. Many parents can tell stories of how sleep patterns changed in their children once the teenage years took a foothold on life and their kids would go to sleep later. And while it is true that social events, homework, sports, television, social media and evening jobs might impact on a teenager's sleep, there is now ample evidence showing us that internal biological processes also influence adolescent sleep.

While melatonin levels appear to change and impact on teenage sleep patterns, serotonin levels also appear to vary during the teenage years. Serotonin is an important chemical for helping us to feel calm and relaxed. It can have an impact on mood fluctuations, anxiety, impulse control and levels of arousal, and low levels of serotonin have been associated with depression, sleep disorders and a variety of behavioural disorders. Some of the latest research available also suggests that serotonin plays a powerful role in moral judgement and decision making, and influences social behaviour. During the teenage years, levels of serotonin can temporarily decline and teenage girls are especially susceptible to lower levels of serotonin given that this neurotransmitter is influenced by oestrogen during the menstrual cycle. High levels of oestrogen enhance levels of serotonin, oxytocin and dopamine, while low levels see corresponding decreases in those chemicals. The potential for low-to-high fluctuations of serotonin during the teenage years has led a number of researchers to speculate that serotonin is complicit in increased impulsivity and greater risks of depression during adolescence.

While serotonin can impact on moods and aspects of behaviour, dopamine is another powerful neurotransmitter that can influence how we feel and act, and it appears to fluctuate markedly during the teenage years. In itself, dopamine is often referred to as the brain's 'pleasure' neurotransmitter, given it plays a role in novelty and reward-seeking behaviours, feelings of wellbeing and motivation. New experiences, especially those associated with some element of risk, thrill or degree of danger, can elevate dopamine and produce feelings of intense pleasure. So influential is dopamine that low levels have been associated with a range of challenges from difficulties maintaining attention on a task to Parkinson's disease, while exceedingly high levels are evident in those who suffer from schizophrenia, Tourette's syndrome and obsessive-compulsive disorder. It should be apparent that levels of this neurotransmitter can have a profound impact on a person.

During the teenage years dopamine levels are at their highest and then begin to decline as adulthood approaches, and this can impact on behaviour, given how dopamine engages the brain's reward systems. So strong is the influence of dopamine in teenagers that neurodevelopmental studies have identified that there seems to be a dopamine 'power play' between the higher-order thinking regions and the more primal emotive systems, resulting in the immature prefrontal cortex of teenagers giving way to the powerful emotions associated with impulsivity and risk-taking. Importantly, while it appears that all teenagers will take part in some measure of risk-taking, there are also individual differences in the chemicals and systems noted above, suggesting that some teenagers will engage in far riskier behaviours than others and this can also be impacted on by the brain's reward systems.

Without going into the fine neuroscientific details of how the brain senses, interprets and mediates rewards, both human and animal studies tell us that the reward system of the brain undergoes massive changes during the teenage years, resulting in greater sensation seeking, reward seeking, and risk-taking behaviours. This change may account for links between teenage risk-taking behaviours and increased mortalities, health-compromising behaviours and harmful outcomes during this time of life. Moreover, changes in behaviour associated with risk-taking, impulsivity and mood swings in teenagers are compounded by all of the other developmental changes noted earlier, and it seems that the teenage brain is primed to do things that might make a six-year-old child cringe in disbelief. It is these types of behaviours and approaches to working with teenagers that are explored next.

UNDERSTANDING AND WORKING WITH TEENAGERS

Understanding teenagers?! Many generations have tried but we can view teenage behaviours differently and develop a better understanding of teenagers if we continually remind ourselves that the teenage brain is a work in progress. From the outset, then, it is important to remind ourselves that teenagers, regardless of physical appearance and size, are not smaller versions of adults. The brain is changing during the teenage years and it is awash with emotion amid a stage of restructuring and, at times, the potential absence of logical reasoning. Emotions can be both positive and negative in terms of teenage behaviour and, as such, behaviour should be seen as a biological symptom as well as a result of social circumstance. Teenagers may do some beguiling things, but this is part of a normal stage of identity formation. From that perspective, *it is important to ensure that boundaries and guidelines are clear, concise and unambiguous. It is also important to foster lines of open communication and carefully temper any teenage need for independence with the experience of an adult* – in this sense mentoring programmes and positive relationships with adults around them are important considerations when working with, and raising, teenagers.

A further consideration lies in recognising that *the teenage brain is primed for sensation seeking and risk-taking activities.* These types of activities will vary according to gender, experience and exposure to a variety of environmental stimuli. Sensation seeking may also occur in the guise of experimentation and *teenagers are particularly susceptible to chemical addictions including to nicotine, alcohol and other drugs.* Whenever possible, *creating opportunities for teenagers to take risks in a positive and pro-social way may assist in providing an environment for them to extend themselves and avoid harmful alternatives.* The key to all of this lies in providing supportive environments that allow teenagers to take risks on various levels and in various contexts. Once again, however, firm boundaries and structures are needed. *Many teenagers take risks through extracurricular activities such as sport and music but it is important to find alternatives for those who don't.* One relatively easy way of accommodating this would be to *develop 'rites of passage' activities that not only allow for the facilitation of pre-arranged elements of risk but also offer opportunities for individuals to recognise and affirm their transition into adulthood.* Teachers, counsellors and parents alike can do this in various contexts and with a variety of positive outcomes.

In understanding that teenagers will engage in risk-taking and sensation seeking, it is also important to remember that *teenagers may not always understand the implications and consequences of their choices and decisions and, as such, talking to and supporting teenagers is important.* However, *it is also important for adults to listen, listen and listen some more and, in doing so, also remember that they were once teenagers as well.* Every generation seems to think the current younger generation is problematic but it turns out that that is not the case and simply a matter of misplaced opinion. Neurologically speaking, current generations of teenagers aren't any different from previous generations and while they live in different times and contexts, they still share a need to be heard with those of us who grew up some years ago. Empathy goes a long way when working with teenagers. Furthermore, there is a common tendency to demonise teenagers in the media and it is not uncommon to see headlines such as 'teens run wild' in newspapers. *Always remember that for every teenager who does something that makes the news in a negative fashion, there are thousands who don't and we should celebrate the teenage years regardless of how many challenges they present.* Showering young people with positives and striving to ensure positive environments goes a long way towards enhancing brain maturation. Cognitive energy channelled in this manner will go much further than trying to find a solution to an arguably unanswerable question such as '*What could they be thinking?*'

Along with being empathetic when needed, *it is also important to model the types of behaviours you expect and to encourage teenagers towards self-regulation. Teenagers do value their peers but we also know that the most significant person in a teenager's life is typically an adult role model,* usually a parent but often a teacher, coach or other adult. Teenage brains are particularly susceptible to emulating the wrong role models and social media can provide far too many of those. Adults need to model the types of behaviours that they want the teenagers around them to emulate, which also helps to build self-regulation in the teenage brain. *A teenager presented with appropriate models for dealing with anger, frustration or other emotions will increasingly become aware of their own behaviour, understand the importance of controlling it when necessary, and display positive approaches to dealing with life's highs and lows.*

Finally, avoid rushing teenagers into maturity or 'growing up'. There is nothing that any adult can do to hurry the natural developmental timelines of the brain. The discussion above has offered broad guidelines towards understanding and working with teenagers but each brain, and each teen, is different. Take hope from any examples of maturation you see and be sure to acknowledge those things that appear to be the actions of a maturing mind. It is equally important to remember that while our understanding of the brain has improved over the years, there are some time-honoured concepts that remain true. *Teenagers respond well to adults who value and love them and they listen to and trust those adults who care about them, avoid judging them and invest time in, and with, them.* The teenage brain is a work in progress and it can be guided to grow emotionally, socially and intellectually in a positive and healthy manner. It just needs time, attention, encouragement, guidance, love and the voices of experience from those who grew through similar times of change, experimentation and self-discovery. In the end, understanding the teenage brain is not just about understanding the young people around us, but in understanding the teenage brain, we are also offered a mechanism for remembering who we once were so that we can now provide the support needed for healthy development. In short, we don't have to just accept the neurodevelopmental changes outlined in this chapter, we can actually shape and change them.

Author biography

Dr Michael Nagel is an Associate Professor at the University of the Sunshine Coast, where he teaches and researches in the areas of cognition, human development, behaviour and learning. He is the author of ten books on child development and learning used by teachers and parents in over twenty countries. Dr Nagel has delivered over 300 workshops and seminars for parents and teachers nationally and internationally. Nominated as Australian Lecturer of the Year each year since 2010, Dr Nagel is a member of the prestigious International Neuropsychological Society, is the Queensland Director of the Australian Council on Children and the Media, and is a feature writer for *Jigsaw* and the *Child* series of magazines which collectively offers parenting advice to more than one million Australian readers.

www.michaelnagel.com.au

See also:

Chapter 18. What is Resilience and How to Do It

Chapter 19: Harnessing the Minecraft Mindset for Success

Chapter 20: Using Positive Psychology

Chapter 21: Food, Mood and Mental Health

Chapter 23: Online Time Management

Recommended websites:

Mumsnet: www.mumsnet.com/teenagers

Relate: www.relate.org.uk/relationship-help/help-family-life-and-parenting/parenting-
teenagers

Further reading:

Blakemore, SJ 2007, 'The social brain of a teenager', *Psychologist*, vol. 20, no. 10, pp
600–602.

Carew, TJ & Magsamen, SH 2010, 'Neuroscience and education: An ideal partnership for
producing evidence-based solutions to guide 21st century learning', Neuron, vol. 67,
no. 5, pp 685–688.

Carskadon, MA 2002, *Adolescent sleep patterns: Biological, social, and psychological influences*,
Cambridge University Press, Cambridge.

Casey, BJ 2013, 'The teenage brain: An overview', *Current Directions in Psychological Science*,
vol. 22, no. 2, pp 80–81.

Chassin, L, Hussong, A & Beltran, I 2009, 'Adolescent substance use' in Lerner, RM &
Steinberg, L (Eds.), *Handbook of adolescent psychology: Volume 1: Individual bases of adolescent
development* (3rd ed), John Wiley & Sons. Inc, Hoboken, pp 723–763.

Dahl, RE 2003, 'Beyond raging hormones: The tinderbox in the teenage brain', *Cerebrum*,
vol. 5, no. 3, pp 7–22.

Feinstein, SG 2009, *Secrets of the teenage brain: Research-based strategies for reaching and teaching
today's adolescents* (2nd Ed), Corwin, Thousand Oaks.

Giedd, J 2010, 'The teen brain: Primed to learn, primed to take risks' in Gordan, D (Ed),
Cerebrum: Emerging ideas in brain science 2010, Dana Press, New York, pp 62–70.

Howard, PJ 2006, *The owner's manual for the brain: Everyday applications from mind-brain research*
(3rd ed), Bard Press, Austin.

Medina, J 2008, *Brain rules: 12 principles for surviving and thriving at work, home and school*, Pear
Press, Seattle, Washington.

Nagel, MC 2009, 'Mind the mind: Understanding the links between stress, emotional
well-being and learning in educational contexts', *The International Journal of Learning*,
vol. 16, no. 2, pp 33–42.

Nagel, MC & Scholes, L 2016, *Understanding development and learning: Implications for teaching*,
Oxford University Press, Melbourne.

Nagel, MC 2014, *In the Middle: The adolescent brain, behaviour and learning*, Australian Council
of Educational Research, Melbourne.

Nagel, MC 2012, *Nurturing a healthy mind: Doing what matters most for your child's developing
brain*, Exisle Publishing, Newcastle.

Ponton, LE 1997, *The romance of risk: Why teenagers do the things they do*, Basic Books, New
York.

Sousa, D 2009, *How the brain influences behaviour,* Corwin Press Inc, Thousand Oaks.

Spear, LP 2010, *The behavioural neuroscience of adolescence,* W.W. Norton & Company, Inc., New York.

Strauch, B 2003, *The primal teen: What the new discoveries about the teenage brain tell us about our kids,* Doubleday, New York.

Walsh, D 2004, *Why do they act that way? A survival guide to the adolescent brain for you and your teen,* Free Press, New York.

 For more online resources visit:
generationnext.com.au/handbook

23. ONLINE TIME MANAGEMENT

Tena Davies

To help young people manage time online, I recommend taking a balanced and collaborative approach. This involves setting boundaries in collaboration with young people and empowering them with tools to help self-manage their time online.

INTRODUCTION

Globally and across Australia, managing a young person's time online can be problematic for parents, with 55 per cent reporting that they attempt to limit their children's amount of time online or restricting what times children can go online. A further 65 per cent report that they have 'digitally grounded' their teen by taking away their mobile phone or internet access.[1]

In my experience working across independent and government schools in Australia, the most pressing issue for parents regarding their children's cyber use is managing their time online. This is not surprising given how frequently young people use the internet, which is estimated to be more than three times per day for most Australian teens aged fourteen to fifteen. This is due in large part to smartphone ownership. Young people are also online late into the night, with 28 per cent of fourteen- to fifteen-year-olds going online after 10 p.m.[2]

What may be surprising, given how much young people resist having their online time restricted by their parents, is that they feel themselves that wasting time online is a major issue. When I survey secondary-school-aged children, they rate wasting time online instead of doing homework or sleeping as the most pressing issue facing them regarding the internet. In my surveys, more than 85 per cent of students typically state that wasting time online interferes with their ability to sleep and do homework. Students rate social media as the biggest time waster, noting that they spend an average of three-plus hours across social media platforms.

The impact of wasting time online is significant. Students report that it leads to them feeling anxious about looming homework. Parents report that attempting to manage their children's time online is a major source of conflict.[3]

HOW TO MANAGE A YOUNG PERSON'S TIME ONLINE

Managing time online is not a simple matter and it is one that will be different in each household. I recommend that families sit down together and discuss how their cyber use is impacting them both positively and negatively across important life domains: friends, family, the internet, school, and any other important areas such as sport. The solutions should aim to reduce the negative aspects of the internet and appreciate and respect the positives that it brings.

Your role as a parent should ideally be to act as a media mentor by providing your child with tools and guidelines to regulate their use. However, it is also important to 'parent' the internet in the same way that you may parent other areas of your child's life, by putting in reasonable boundaries and moderate consequences if your child is not displaying good self-regulating skills.

When discussing your child's internet use, make sure to keep an open mind. The digital world is an important source of social contact for young people. They use the internet to maintain and extend relationships with their peers. When we were growing up we used to talk on the phone or hang out at the local café. Nowadays, social media is the virtual hangout. Therefore, spending time online represents an important way of connecting with peers but it does need to be managed. The expression 'fire is a good servant and a poor master' also applies to internet use.

A CASE STUDY

Rose and Tom were frustrated with their children's cyber use. It seemed that they were always either on their smartphones or iPads. Claire, aged twelve, went to bed with her iPhone under the guise that she needed it as an alarm in the morning. Carl, sixteen, was about to start GCSEs and seemed to be playing online games more and more frequently. He played online games in his room and often went to bed after midnight.

Rose and Tom had tried a number of things to attempt to manage their children's cyber use. They 'grounded' Claire and Carl frequently but this seemed to make things worse and escalated into screaming fights. They would try to take their children's devices from them but this never lasted long and led to family discord. Rose and Tom tried to reason with their children, explaining why their online use was bad for them. Each had practically begged their children to stop using their devices late at night. Often they put in place consequences such as no media for a week, but this was impossible to enforce.

When they came to my office they were at a loss as to what to do and asked if I could please try to reason with their children. I noticed that they were stuck in a cycle of escalating consequences.

What struck me about this case was that although Rose and Tom were competent parents, they didn't seem to 'parent' their children's cyber use in the way they would other areas of their children's life. Instead, they pleaded with their children to be more sensible. They swung between being overly permissive with their children's cyber use (playing video games and playing on phones late at night) and being overly authoritarian by putting in place harsh consequences, which invariably led to fighting and which they didn't stick to anyway.

As a first step, I asked the family to come in for a meeting.

I asked the family how spending time online helps them achieve their goals across important areas of their life including friendships, friends, family, school and health. I also asked how their cyber use was negatively impacting each area of life.

The kids noted that it was useful to use the internet to connect with their peers and do some of their homework. They also noted that they probably spent too much time on social media and that after a certain point it was *not* useful, especially late at night. Claire noted that spending time too much time online kept her from exercising, which was important to her. Rose and Tom noted they both spent too much time playing on their own phones and too much time fighting about the internet as a family. I asked each family member to come up with a few guidelines to address the issues.

Claire said she would do all of her homework before catching up with her friends online, but predictably this only lasted one day. Carl said he wouldn't fight with his parents but that lasted less than one day! I find that this is common with young people, who sometimes devise well-intended and idealistic solutions that are difficult to implement.

After their initial attempts, over the course of a few weeks I met up with Rose and Tom as well as the family as a whole. I met with the parents to give them tools to 'parent' their children's cyber use. I also made some suggestions for Carl and Claire to experiment with so that they could learn to self-regulate their cyber use.

In the end, we focused on a few simple things. The first was to ensure that cyber use did not interfere with sleep, academic achievement and important family time. The family agreed as a whole to no screen time during family mealtimes, which were about thirty minutes' duration. The second was to stop using devices at 10 p.m. and wind down for sleep. The trade-off for this for the kids was that the parents would respect their need to connect with peers and have fun online. The rules would also be relaxed during the school holidays. Finally, and this took more work, the kids agreed to use productivity software to ensure their homework got done three nights a week. Carl, who played multiplayer games, agreed to three no-game nights provided he wasn't 'nagged' about it on other nights. Each child also agreed to undertake one face-to-face activity. Claire started taking a yoga class after school that she also followed on Instagram and Carl joined the local gym.

With Carl and Claire, I worked through what they thought was a fair consequence for non-compliance. They said that if they didn't hand over their phone at 10 p.m. they had to hand it over an hour earlier the next night. They also said that if their grades slipped they knew they would have to revisit their agreement.

Following are some points for managing cyber use with adolescents:

- **Start by asking them how the internet is both enhancing and hindering their life** in important areas such as friends, family, relationships, and their health and wellbeing. Then see if your solutions can reduce the negatives without significantly compromising the positives. An example would be handing over the phone to parents at 10 p.m. on weeknights during the school term so that they can prepare for sleep. This gives them ample time to socialise before going off the grid. Ensure the solution is sensible, workable and one that can be enforced.
- **Aim for reasonable use:** ask them what they think this is. My experience is that young people usually suggest something idealistic such as using it for one hour after doing their homework. Unfortunately, this is not realistic. However, asking them what they think is a good way of engaging them and getting the ball rolling. When adolescents suggest an unrealistic amount of screen time, I help them to work out a more realistic solution together.
- **Aim for incremental change:** if your child has until now stayed online until midnight, saying 'no screen time after 8 p.m.' may not work. Instead, wind it down one or two hours. Then reassess.

- **Focus on time offline rather than restricting time online:** think about what times are important to be away from technology. The times I think are important are family mealtimes and an hour or so before bed as this assists with winding down to go to sleep.
- **Have periods where rules are more flexible:** relax rules on weekends and also school holidays and, if possible, even some weeknights. This makes for fewer fights but it also makes for more compliant kids.
- **Balance time online with offline activities:** a great way to get your child offline is ensure they are engaged in an offline activity such as sport or another hobby. Team sports are particularly good because they are active and it teaches them social skills to interact in a group.
- **Model the behaviour you want to see:** how often do you go to a cafe and see couples and families playing on their phone rather than connecting with each other? It's very common that we are slaves to our devices. However, it's difficult to enforce rules if we are not ourselves living by them. If you want your child to talk to you during dinner, leave your phone away from the dinner table.
- **Focus on the big issues:** sleep loss is a common issue for adolescents. They tend to go to bed late and wake up early to go to school. Sleep loss has a number of consequences. In addition to young people being tired, poor sleep leads to difficulty with concentration, memory and their ability to learn. This in turn leads to worse outcomes for their learning.[4]
- **Give small consequences rather than issuing big threats:** agree with your child two or three consequences for non-compliance. Make sure they are limited to one day. For example, for the rule *no phone after 10 p.m.*, if they give you the phone late, deduct that time from the next day.
- **Have as few rules as possible (within reason):** aim to have no more than three or so rules about cyber use. The rules

I highly recommend are: no screen time thirty minutes before bed; no playing violent online games (or at least limiting this significantly on weekdays); and using productivity software to get work done.

- **A little less conversation, a little more action:** one of the unhelpful behaviours many of us engage in (myself included) is spending too much time trying to reason with children. We often start off reasonably and end up lecturing or worse. We might say something like: 'We discussed this yesterday and we agreed that you are not to go to bed with your phone. I'm really disappointed in you, if you keep this up I'll cancel your mobile plan and you won't have a phone at all! I should never have bought you a phone. You are so ungrateful!' Notice how as the 'reasoning' goes on it escalates and also notice how there is no consequence, just a lecture and an often empty threat. A better way to go is to agree a consequence with a child for non-compliance of a rule ahead of time, then enforce the consequence when needed without a lecture. It would look something like this: 'Claire, we discussed and agreed that you give me your phone at 10 p.m. It's 10.15 p.m. and you are still on it. Please give me your phone. As discussed, your consequence is that tomorrow night you need to give me your phone 15 minutes early.' Then take the phone and walk out. No conversation, just action. Be sure to follow through the next night. The fewer the consequences, the better.

- **Implement a no-screen night.** Whether once a week or once a month, having a technology-free night is a great way to reconnect (pardon the pun) with the family. Be sure that you plan something fun like going for a walk or out for ice cream, or stay in and play board games. Reflect on how the night went and try to implement on a smaller scale at other times (i.e. the *hour of no power* twice a week).

TIPS FOR ADOLESCENTS

- **Use technology to self-regulate time online.** There are many types of productivity software available to download as apps onto smartphones and laptops. The one I use is called Focus Keeper but there are many other types available. A search on Google/Google Play/iPhone app store will reveal many options.
- **One thing at a time.** Alternate blocks of work with blocks of socialising. While it would be a good idea to do all your homework before socialising, it may not suit you. If that doesn't suit, spend some time doing only homework and then spend another period of time socialising. Trying to do both means that you won't be able to do either well. You can alternate 30 minutes of work with 15 minutes of socialising. You'll still get more work done than if you try to multitask.

DON'TS FOR PARENTS

Don't set rules you can't enforce. While it may be tempting to say things like 'Don't get a [insert latest social media craze] account', the reality is that your child is likely to do it anyway. Instead of saying, 'Don't get Snapchat', discuss some conduct rules and ensure they are using their privacy settings appropriately. I'd rather say yes and be involved in setting parameters than say no and have the behaviour go underground where I'd have no influence.

Don't set yourself up for a fight. If you go in frustrated, saying something like 'Why are you still on your phone? You are such a problem!' this makes your young person either tune out or respond in kind. Instead, set up a time to talk when you are both calm.

Don't have too many rules. When rules go on and on, adhering to them becomes difficult. I'd have a limited number of rules and one or two consequences for non-compliance instead.

Don't be digitally clueless. One of the things I hear most when working with young people is that their parents have no idea about their cyber world. The problem with this is that it is very difficult to parent what you don't know. So my advice is be on whatever your children are using so that you can have meaningful conversations with your child about it. After all, good teaching starts with learning your subject matter.

FREQUENTLY ASKED QUESTIONS

I can't take my child's phone away from them at night because they need it as an alarm to wake them up in the morning.
Getting enough sleep is essential for your child's mental health, wellbeing and ability to learn. Viewing bright visual displays at night increases alertness and does not set them up for sleep.

If they need an alarm, buy them one. The sleep battle is one worth fighting.

I can't get my child offline late at night because they are doing homework. Is there anything I should do?
Chances are your child is doing homework at 11.30 p.m. because they were too busy socialising online earlier in the evening. I'd negotiate with your young person about how they might start homework earlier in the night. For example, by doing 30 minutes of homework as soon as they get home to get things rolling. Then they can alternate work blocks and social blocks. Often once they start they will be less prone to procrastinate throughout the night. Productivity software may also help (Google will reveal many options). It may also be useful to speak to your child's year level coordinator to determine how much homework they have and how much they need the internet for this.

My child plays multiplayer games that go for hours. How can they balance this and their studies?
This is certainly a challenging one. What I'd suggest is that they have alternating game and non-game nights. This way they can enjoy their gaming and also their studies. If they prove that they are unable to balance this in a reasonable way, I would consider banning the games during the week over the school term.

WHEN TO WORRY

I think the biggest red flag is a significant change of behaviour and a child who withdraws from life. For example, if a child who regularly used social media to connect with peers suddenly says she is closing all of her accounts, this may indicate something is wrong. This suggests that they have had an adverse experience, such as bullying. Or a child who previously loved sport now spends most of his time in his room playing a multiplayer game. If you find yourself saying, 'They used to play soccer/love music/spend time with the family', that's a sign that they may be withdrawing from life. Have a calm conversation with your young person or seek professional advice from a registered Adolescent Psychologist. See British Psychological Society (www.bps.org.uk), to find a trained psychologist in your area.

Author biography

Tena Davies is a Melbourne-based psychologist and cyber expert. She has recently completed a Clinical Psychology Master's degree with a thesis on parenting the internet. She works with young people and families to help support a young person's cyber wellness. Her approach to working with young people and families is to promote a balanced and practical approach.

www.tenadavies.com

See also:
Chapter 22: Understanding the Teenage Brain

Recommended websites:
Pew Research Center: www.pewinternet.org
US National Sleep Foundation: www.sleepfoundation.org
UK Sleep Council: sleepcouncil.org.uk

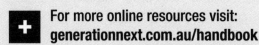

For more online resources visit:
generationnext.com.au/handbook

ENDNOTES

2. What to do in a Mental Health Crisis

1. Jorm, A.F., Korten, A.E., Jacomb, P.A., Christensen, H., Rodgers, B. & Pollitt, P., '"Mental health literacy": a survey of the public's ability to recognise mental disorders and their beliefs about the effectiveness of treatment.' *Medical Journal of Australia*, 166, 1997, pp. 182–186.

2. Hadlaczky, G., Hokby, S., Mkrtchian, A., Carli, V. & Wasserman, D., 'Mental Health First Aid is an effective public health intervention for improving knowledge, attitudes, and behaviour: A meta-analysis.' *International Review of Psychiatry*, 4, 2014, pp. 467–475.

3. Kelly, C.M., Kitchener, B.A., & Jorm, A.F., *Youth Mental Health First Aid: A Manual for Adults Assisting Young People* (4th ed), Melbourne: Mental Health First Aid Australia; 2017. (Previously unpublished data from the 2007 National Survey of Mental Health and Wellbeing.)

4. Lawrence. D., Johnson, S., Hakefost, J., Boterhoven De Haan, K., Sawyer, M., Ainley, J., & Zubrick, S.R., *The Mental Health of Children and Adolescents. Report on the Second Australian Child and Adolescent Survey of Mental Health and Wellbeing*. Canberra: Department of Health; 2015.

5. Australian Bureau of Statistics, *2007 National Survey of Mental Health and Wellbeing: Summary of Results. (Document 4326.0)*. Canberra: ABS; 2008.

6. Fischer, J.A., Kelly, C.M., Kitchener, B.A. & Jorm, A.F., 'Development of Guidelines for Adults on How to Communicate With Adolescents About Mental Health Problems and Other Sensitive Topics', *Sage Open*, 2013, 3 (4). Mental Health First Aid Australia, *Communicating with adolescents: guidelines for adults on how to communicate with adolescents about mental health problems and other sensitive topics*. Melbourne: Mental Health First Aid Australia, 2014.

7. Langlands, R.L., Jorm, A.F., Kelly, C.M. & Kitchener, B.A., 'First aid for depression: A Delphi consensus study with consumers, carers and clinicians', *Journal of Affective Disorders*, 105, 2008, pp. 157–165. Mental Health First Aid Australia, *Depression: first aid guidelines*. Melbourne: Mental Health First Aid Australia, 2008.

6. Understanding Self-harm

1. Martin, G., Swannell, S., Harrison, J., Hazell, P., & Taylor, A., *The Australian National Epidemiological Study of Self-Injury (ANESSI),* Centre for Suicide Prevention Studies, Brisbane, Australia, 2010.

2. Martin, G., Swannell, S., Harrison, J., Hazell, P., & Taylor, A., *The Australian National Epidemiological Study of Self-Injury (ANESSI),* Centre for Suicide Prevention Studies, Brisbane, Australia, 2010.

3. Klonsky, E.D., May, A.M. & Glenn, C.R., 'The relationship between nonsuicidal self-injury and attempted suicide: Converging evidence from four samples,' *Journal of Abnormal Psychology*, 122, 2013, pp. 231–237.

4. Ross, A.M., Jorm, A.F. & Kelly, C.M., 'Re-development of mental health first aid guidelines for deliberate non-suicidal self-injury: A Delphi study', *BMC Psychiatry*, 14, 2014, Aug 19; pp. 236.

7. Suicide and Attempted Suicide

1. Lawrence, D., Johnson, S., Hakefost, J., Boterhoven De Haan, K., Sawyer, M., Ainley, J. & Zubrick, S.R., *The Mental Health of Children and Adolescents. Report on the Second Australian Child and Adolescent Survey of Mental Health and Wellbeing*, Canberra, Department of Health, 2015.

2. Johnston, A.K., Pirkis, J.E. & Burgess, P.M., *Suicidal thoughts and behaviours among Australian adults: findings from the 2007 National Survey of Mental Health and Wellbeing, Australian & New Zealand Journal of Psychiatry*, 2009, 43, pp. 635–43.

3. Ross, A.M., Kelly, C.M. & Jorm, A.F., 'Re-development of mental health first aid guidelines for suicidal ideation and behaviour: a Delphi study', *BMC Psychiatry*, 2014; 14: 1.

8. Towards Prevention: Understanding Child Sexual Assault

1. Finkelhor, D., 'The international epidemiology of child sexual abuse.' *Child Abuse and Neglect*, 18, 1994, pp. 409–417; James, M., *Child abuse and neglect: Redefining the issues* (Trends and Issues Series, No. 146), Canberra, Australia: Australian Institute of Criminology, 2000; Queensland Crime Commission & Queensland Police Service, Project Axis, Volume 1: Child sexual abuse in Queensland: The nature and extent. Brisbane: Queensland Crime Commission, 2000.

2. Gilbert, R., Spatz-Widom, C., Browne, K., Fergusson, D., Webb E. & Janson, S., 'Burden and consequences of child maltreatment in high income countries', *The Lancet,* 373(9657), 2009, pp. 68–81.

3. Beitchman, J.H., Zucker, K.J., Hood, J.E., DaCosta, D., & Akaman D., 'A review of the short-term effects of child sexual abuse', *Journal of Abuse and Neglect*, 15, 1991, pp. 537–556; Browne, K. & Lynch, M., 1994. 'Prevention: Actions speak louder than words', *Child Abuse Review*, 3, 1994, pp. 241–244.

4. Abdulrehman, R. Y., & De Luca, R. V., 'The implications of childhood sexual abuse on adult social behaviour', *Journal of Family Violence*, 16 (2), 2001, pp. 1573–2851; Alaggia, R., 'Disclosing the trauma of child sexual abuse: A gender analysis', *Journal of Loss and Trauma*, 10, 2005, pp. 453–470; Jonzon, E., & Lindblad, F., 'Disclosure, reactions, and social support: findings from a sample of adult victims of child sexual abuse', *Child Maltreatment*, 9 (2), 2004, pp. 190–200; Orsoli, L., Kia-Keating, M., & Grossman, F. K., 'I keep that hush-hush: Male survivors of sexual abuse and the challenges of disclosure', *Journal of Counselling Psychology*, 55 (3), 2008, pp. 333–345.

5. National Child Protection Clearinghouse, *Child Abuse Prevention Resource Sheet* (no. 7), 2005.

6. Kogan, S.M., 'Disclosing unwanted sexual experiences: results from a national survey of adolescent women', *Child Abuse and Neglect*, 28, 2004, pp. 147–165.

7. National Child Protection Clearinghouse, *Child Abuse Prevention Resource Sheet* (no. 7), 2005.

8. Kogan, S.M., 'Disclosing unwanted sexual experiences: results from a national survey of adolescent women', *Child Abuse and Neglect*, 28, 2004, pp. 147–165.

9. Smallbone, S. & Wortley, R. (2000), *Child sexual abuse in Queensland: Offender characteristics and modus operandi*, Brisbane [Qld]: Queensland Crime Commission.

10. Lanning, K., *Child Molesters: A Behavioural Analysis* (5th ed), Alexandria [Va.]: National Center for Missing and Exploited Children, 2010.

11. Finkelhor, D., *Child Sexual Abuse: New theory and research*, New York [NY]: The Free Press, 1984.

12. Leclerc, B., Proulx, J. & McKibben, A., 'Modus operandi of sexual offenders working or doing voluntary work with children and adolescents', *Journal of Sexual Aggression*, 11(2), 2005, pp. 187–195.

13. Jensen, T. K., Gulbrandsen, W., Mossige, S., Reichelt, S. & Tjersland, O. A., 'Reporting possible sexual abuse: A qualitative study on children's perspectives and the context for disclosure', *Child Abuse and Neglect*, 29, 12, 2005, pp. 1395–1413.

14. Crisma, M., Bascelli, E., Paci, D., & Romito, R., 'Adolescents who experienced sexual abuse: Fears, needs and impediments to disclosure', *Child Abuse and Neglect*, 28, 2004, pp. 1035–1048.

15. Alaggia, R. & Kirshenbaum, S., 'Speaking the unspeakable: Exploring the impact of family dynamics on child sexual abuse disclosures', *Families in Society*, 856, 2005, pp. 227–234.

16. Paine, M.L. & Hansen, D.J., 'Factors influencing children to self-disclose sexual abuse', *Clinical Psychology Review*, 22, 2002, pp. 271–295.

17. Bhave, S. & Mashanker, V., 'Sexual abuse in children and adolescents'. In S. Gupte (ed.) *Recent Advances in Pediatrics* (Special Volume 17), 2006, pp. 268–290. Daryaganj [India]: Jaypee Brothers Medical Publishers.

18. Elliot, A. & Carnes, C., 'Reactions of nonoffending parents to the sexual abuse of their child: A review of the literature', *Child Maltreatment,* 6(4), 2001, pp. 314–331.

19. Beitchman, J.H., Zucker, K.J., Hood, J.E., DaCosta, D., Akaman D. & Cassavia, E., 'A review of the long term effects of child sexual abuse', *Child Abuse and Neglect,* 16, 1992, pp. 101–118; Briere, J. & Elliott, D., 'Immediate and Long-Term Impacts of Child Sexual Abuse', *The Future of Children,* 4(2), 1994, pp. 54–69.

20. Elliot, A. & Carnes, C., 'Reactions of nonoffending parents to the sexual abuse of their child: A review of the literature', *Child Maltreatment,* 6(4), 2001, pp. 314–331; Wyatt, G. E. & Mickey, M. R., 'Ameliorating the effects of child sexual abuse: an exploratory study of support by parents and others', *Journal of Interpersonal Violence,* 2, 1987, pp. 403–414.

21. Hanson, R.K., Gordon, A., Harris, A.J.R., Marques, J.K., Murphy, W., Quinsey, V.L. & Seto, M.C., 'First report of the collaborative outcome data project on the effectiveness of psychological treatment for sex offenders', *Sexual Abuse: A Journal of Research and Treatment,* 14(2), 2002, pp. 169–194.

22. National Child Protection Clearinghouse, *Child Abuse Prevention Resource Sheet* (no. 7), 2005.

23. Australian Institute of Criminology, *Second Conference on Violence,* June 1993.

24. Wyatt, G. E. & Mickey, M. R., 'Ameliorating the effects of child sexual abuse: an exploratory study of support by parents and others', *Journal of Interpersonal Violence,* 2, 1987, pp. 403–414.

25. Finkelhor, D., *Child Sexual Abuse: New theory and research,* New York [NY]: The Free Press, 1984.

26. Briggs, F., *From Victim to Offender: How child sexual abuse victims become offenders,* St Leonards [NSW]: Allen & Unwin, 1995.

27. Dympna House, *Info Kit: A booklet on childhood sexual abuse,* Haberfield [NSW]: Dympna House, 1998.

28. Jensen, T. K., Gulbrandsen, W., Mossige, S., Reichelt, S. & Tjersland, O. A., 'Reporting possible sexual abuse: A qualitative study on children's perspectives and the context for disclosure', *Child Abuse and Neglect,* 29, 12, 2005, pp. 1395–1413.

10. Supporting a Young Person in their Decision not to Use Alcohol or Other Drugs

1. Bailey, V., Baker, A-M., Cave, L., Fildes, J., Perrens, B., Plummer, J. & Wearring, A., *Mission Australia's 2016 Youth Survey Report,* Mission Australia, 2016.

2. White, V. & Williams, T., *Australian secondary school students' use of tobacco, alcohol, and over-the-counter and illicit substances in 2014,* Cancer Council Victoria, 2016.

3. Herring, R., Bayley, M. & Hurcombe, R., '"But no one told me it's okay to not drink": A qualitative study of young people who drink little or no alcohol', *Journal of Substance Use,* 19, 2014, pp. 95–102.

4. Nairn, K., Higgins, J., Thompson, B., Anderson, M. & Fu, N., '"It's Just Like the Teenage Stereotype, You Go Out and Drink and Stuff": Hearing from Young People who Don't Drink', *Journal of Youth Studies* 9, 2006, pp. 287–304.

5. ibid.

6. Herring, R., Bayley, M. & Hurcombe, R., '"But no one told me it's okay to not drink": A qualitative study of young people who drink little or no alcohol', *Journal of Substance Use,* 19, 2014, pp. 95–102.

16. Bigorexia: Muscle Dysmorphia in Young People

1. Cafri, G., Olivarida, R. & Thompson, J., 'Symptom Characteristics and Psychiatric Comorbidity Among Males With Muscle Dysmorphia', *Comprehensive Psychiatry,* 49, 2008, pp. 374–379.; Hitzeroth et al., 2001; Olivardia et al., 2000.

2. Olivardia R., Pope H.G., Jr, & Hudson J.I., '"Muscle dysmorphia" in male weightlifters: A case-control study', *American Journal of Psychiatry,* 157, 2000, pp. 1291–1296.

19. Harnessing the Minecraft Mindset for Success

1. Brand, J., & Todhunter, S., Digital Australia 2016

2. www.people.hofstra.edu/Jeffrey_J_Froh/spring 2010 web/ELYS_FINAL PROOF.pdf

3. www.schlechtycenter.org/about-the-center

4. Munns, G., Sawyer, W., & Cole, B. (Eds.), *Exemplary teachers of students in poverty,* Routledge, 2013.

5. Geirland, John, 'Go With The Flow', *Wired* magazine, September, Issue 4.09, 1996.

6. www.ncbi.nlm.nih.gov/pubmed/11392867

7. Check out planetminecraft.com for more ideas.

23. Online Time Management

1. 'Parents, teens, and digital monitoring', 2016, www.pewinternet.org

2. 'Aussie teens and kids online', ACMA, 2016, www.acma.gov.au/theacma/engage-blogs/research-snapshots/aussie-teens-and-kids-online

3. 'Parents, teens, and digital monitoring', 2016, www.pewinternet.org

4. 'Teens and Sleep', National Sleep Foundation, 2016, www.sleepfoundation.org/sleep-topics/teens-and-sleep

THE MENTAL STILLNESS APP

Every year Mission Australia conducts its large survey of Australia's young people to identify their major concerns. Over the past several years the issue of stress has featured high on the list of issues that young people feel they need help with. While everyone might experience periods of stress from time to time, prolonged stress and even sometimes extreme stress for short periods are often precursors for more serious mental health problems. So stress is really something that we ought to help young people manage, and it is something that young people want and need help with.

Over the past decade meditation and mindfulness have become increasingly fashionable as ways of reducing stress, improving mood and generally enhancing wellbeing. To better understand meditation, our research has focused on the ancient ideas from which these practices have arisen. We have found that one relatively less known part of the meditation tradition, the experience of mental silence, is in fact particularly important. This is because clinical trials have consistently shown that the mental silence component of meditation yields stress reducing and mental wellbeing enhancing benefits that are significantly greater than placebo.

Why is mental silence so important? As we each grow more aware of our inner environment, many of us have come to realise that there is a constant 'background mental chatter' that seems to accompany us virtually wherever we go, whatever we do. While we all seem to accept it as a normal part of our inner life mental health professionals also recognise that this 'rumination' can often have a major impact on how we think and feel. In fact the ruminations can themselves both worsen, as well as be the source of, stress. Often, during times of mental illness, these ruminations can become overwhelmingly negative.

Meditation, particularly mental silence, is aimed at specifically addressing this mental noise and its toxic effects on our wellbeing. During the mental silence experience, that inner noise is neutralised and yet the meditator is fully alert, fully aware and in full control of themselves and their faculties, and can think if they want to; however, for the duration of their meditation session they experience no unnecessary mental activity. This is 'mental stillness' or 'mental silence'. It is inherently refreshing, destressing and at the same time energising.

The experience of mental silence, we have found, is specifically associated with beneficial effects on mental and sometimes even physical health. Studies conducted by researchers from Sydney University found that in schools, just 5 to 10 minutes of practice, once or twice a day, was enough to improve mental health and reduce the risk of mental illness. Teachers also reported improved engagement and better mood and associated behaviours in those children who engaged with the techniques.

To make this important method more available, we have developed The Mental Stillness App. This is a free, evidence-based resource that is available to the public, professionals and also to young people. It provides simple guided-meditation sequences on video that can be used on demand. These sequences have been developed over several years of rigorous research and testing. They can be used by anyone from age five to ninety-five.

Find out more about the research and evidence at
www.mentalstillness.org

Kabir Sattarshetty
Kabir is a registered nurse. His research and development of the mental stillness guided meditation sequences was done under the auspices of the Department of Psychiatry, Sydney University, as part of his Masters of Medicine degree.